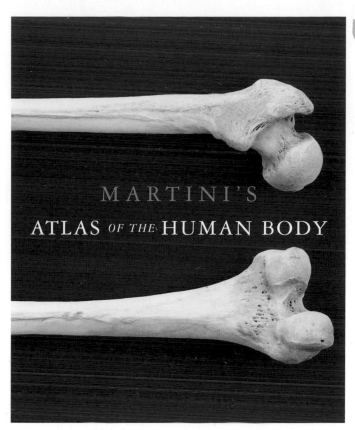

MARTINI'S
ATLAS *OF THE* HUMAN BODY

by

FREDERIC H. MARTINI, PH.D.
University of Hawaii at Manoa

with

WILLIAM C. OBER, M.D.
Art Coordinator and Illustrator

KATHLEEN WELCH
Clinical Consultant

CLAIRE W. GARRISON, R.N.
Illustrator

RALPH T. HUTCHINGS, PH.D.
Biomedical Photographer

Benjamin Cummings

Boston Columbus Indianapolis New York San Francisco Upper Saddle River
Amsterdam Cape Town Dubai London Madrid Milan Munich Paris Montréal Toronto
Delhi Mexico City São Paulo Sydney Hong Kong Seoul Singapore Taipei Tokyo

Executive Editor: Leslie Berriman
Project Editor: Robin Pille
Director of Development: Barbara Yien
Editorial Assistant: Nicole McFadden
Senior Managing Editor: Deborah Cogan
Production Project Manager: Caroline Ayres

Production Management and Composition: S4Carlisle Publishing Services
Interior Designer: Emily Friel
Cover Designer: Yvo Riezebos
Photo Researcher: Maureen Spuhler
Senior Manufacturing Buyer: Stacey Weinberger
Marketing Manager: Derek Perrigo

Cover Photo Credit: PAL 3.0, Pearson Science.

Many of the designations used by manufacturers and sellers to distinguish their products are claimed as trademarks. Where those designations appear in this book, and the publisher was aware of a trademark claim, the designations have been printed in initial caps or all caps.

Photo Credits: 1a, b, 2b, 3c, d, 4a–c, 5a–f, 7a–d, 8a–d, 9a–c, 10, 11a, c, 12a, 14a–d, 15a, c, 16a–c, 18a–c, 19, 20a, 21a–e, 22a–c, 23a, b, 24a, d, 25, 26a, b, 27d, 28, 29a–c, 31, 32, 33b, d, 34a–d, 35a, b, e, f, 36a, b, 37b, 38a, d–f, 39c, 40b, 41a, 42a, b, 43a–d, 44a, b, 45b, d, 46a, b, 49b–e, 51a–d, 52, 53a, 54a–c, 55a, b, 57a, b, 60a, b, 61a–61c, 63, 64, 65, 66, 68b, c, 70a, b, 72a, 73a, b, 74, 75a–d, 76b, 77, 79a, b, 80a, b, 81b, 82b, 83a, b, 84a, b, 85b, 86a, b, 87b, 88b, 89, 90a, b Ralph T. Hutchings 2a, 13f, 23c, 35c, 35g, 38b, 78a Patrick M. Timmons/Michael J. Timmons 3a, 17, 27a–c, 30, 33c, 36, 37a, 39a, d, 40a, 68a, 69a, 76a, 81a, 82a, 87a Mentor Networks, Inc. 6 Image provided by The Digital Cadaver™ Project, courtesy of Visible Productions, Inc. 11b, 12b–d, 13b–e, 20b, 56a–c, 58a–c, 72b, 78b–g, 86c, 87c Frederic H. Martini, Inc. 13a, Pat Lynch/Photo Researchers, Inc. 13g, 24c, 33a, 39b, 54d, 59, 69b, 85a Custom Medical Stock Photo, Inc. 15b, 53c Brendon G. Tillman/Naval Medical Center San Diego 35d ThiemVerlagsgruppe 38c, 47a–d, 49a, 62a, b Pearson Education, PH College 42c, 44c Wellcome Trust Medical 42d, 67 CNRI/Science Photo Library/Photo Researchers, Inc. Researchers, Inc. 45a David York/Medichrome/The Stock Shop, Inc. 48b Marconi Medical Systems, Inc. 48c, 50a, 71b, 78i www.NetAnatomy.com 50b S. Adhikari, et al. The Internet Journal of Surgery. 2008 16:1 50c, 53d Christopher J. Bodin, M. D., Tulane University Medical Center 53c Barry Slaven/P. Mode Photography/Photo Researchers, Inc. 53e P.M. Motta, A. Caggiati, G. Macchiarelli/ Science Photo Library/Photo Researchers, Inc. 45c Science Photo Library/Photo Researchers, Inc. Researchers, Inc. 56d–f, 58d–f Visible Human Project/National Institutes of Health, National Library of Medicine 71a Erin Pheil/iStockphoto 78h Michael L. Richardson; University of Washington of School of Medicine, Dept. of Radiology; www.rad.washington.edu

Library of Congress Cataloging-in-Publication Data

Martini, Frederic.
    Martini's atlas of the human body/by Frederic H. Martini; with William C. Ober, art coordinator and illustrator... [et al.].—9th ed.
        p. ; cm.
    Atlas of the human body
    ISBN: 978-0-321-72456-4
    1. Human anatomy—Atlases. I. Ober, William C. II. Title III. Title: Atlas of the human body
    [DNLM: 1. Anatomy—Atlases. 2. Physiology—Atlases. QS 17]
    QM25.M286 2012
    611—dc22   2010040165

Benjamin Cummings
is an imprint of

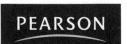

www.pearsonhighered.com

1 2 3 4 5 6 7 8 9 10-DOW-14 13 12 11 10

ISBN 10: 0-321-72456-9 (Student Edition)
ISBN 13: 978-0-321-72456-4 (Student Edition)
ISBN 10: 0-13-249243-1 (NASTA Replacement Edition)
ISBN 13: 978-0-13-249243-0 (NASTA Replacement Edition)

For students in an introductory level anatomy and physiology course, an interpretive anatomical illustration is often the best way to introduce important information without distracting clutter. However, for true understanding, it is important to relate that interpretive view to "real world" anatomy, which is usually much more complex. For example, it is easier to learn the distribution of the major arteries in images that show only arterial and skeletal structures, and yet the concepts learned in that way can be hard to apply and interpret when dealing with a cadaver dissection or a hospital emergency. You might initially think that the best solution would be for a textbook to present illustrations in pairs—an interpretive drawing in conjunction with a matching "real" view such as a cadaver photo or medical scan. In fact, that is how many figures in my textbooks are organized. But to do that globally, for all structures and all systems, would be impractical and unwieldy. First of all, the same photographs would have to appear multiple times—the same image of the dissection of the forearm, for instance, would be paired with illustrations dealing with the bones, muscles, nerves, arteries, veins, and lymphatics of the forearm. Even if this redundancy were tolerable, the textbook would double in length unless the illustrations were reduced in size by half—an unacceptable option because larger images enhance understanding.

This *Atlas* solves that dilemma and makes it easy to relate clear diagrammatic illustrations in the textbook to the real world of dissection images and medical scans. It has been designed to supplement the anatomical illustrations in Martini/Nath/Bartholomew *Fundamentals of Anatomy & Physiology*, Ninth Edition. Figure captions in that textbook indicate the related numbered plates in this *Atlas*. Together, that textbook and this *Atlas* provide a comprehensive and highly-visual orientation to the anatomy of the human body. Because it contains such a comprehensive series of images, this *Atlas* is also a useful companion for my other textbooks, including: Martini/Ober/Nath *Visual Anatomy & Physiology;* Martini/Timmons/Tallitsch *Human Anatomy;* Martini/Bartholomew *Essentials of Anatomy & Physiology;* and Martini/Nath *Anatomy & Physiology*—all available from Pearson Benjamin Cummings.

The images in this *Atlas* are regionally organized. In key areas of the body, diagnostic medical images are paired with cadaver views. This will help students take an additional step—first from the diagrammatic illustration (in the textbook) to a cadaver dissection in a laboratory setting, and then from that inert cadaver to a medical image of a living person. The Contents also includes three quick reference guides for bones, clinical/diagnostic scans, and soft tissue anatomy.

This *Atlas* also contains a visual summary of human embryological development. The timing and depth of coverage of this topic vary widely across classrooms; some instructors cover the embryological development of individual body systems as they discuss each system, whereas others use the topic to wrap up the end of the course, or address the topic briefly only at the beginning and end of the course. There is general agreement, however, that understanding the key events in anatomical development requires an ability to visualize events happening in three-dimensional space. So in the Embryology Summary section of the *Atlas*, we have created a visual presentation that pairs each written description with interpretive art. Students and instructors can refer to the sub-sections in the Embryology Summary, identified by topic and body system, as needed as your course proceeds.

In the preparation of this *Atlas* I have been very fortunate to work with Ralph Hutchings, considered by many to be the world's preeminent anatomical photographer, and Dr. William Ober and Ms. Claire Garrison, superb and creative medical illustrators who worked with me on the complexities of labeling the plates and helped create the Embryology Summaries. I would also like to thank the instructors who contacted me over the last three years with suggestions for the reorganization and improvement of this *Atlas*.

I hope you find this *Atlas* useful. If you have comments or suggestions for improvement, please contact me at the address below.

Frederic H. Martini
martini@maui.net

Contents

Embryology Summaries

Quick Reference Guide to Soft Tissue Anatomy

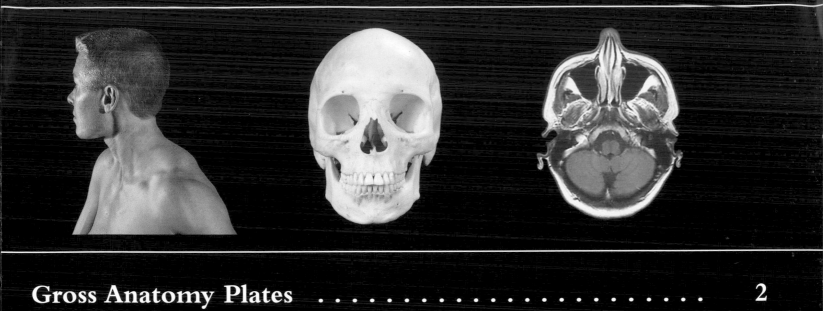

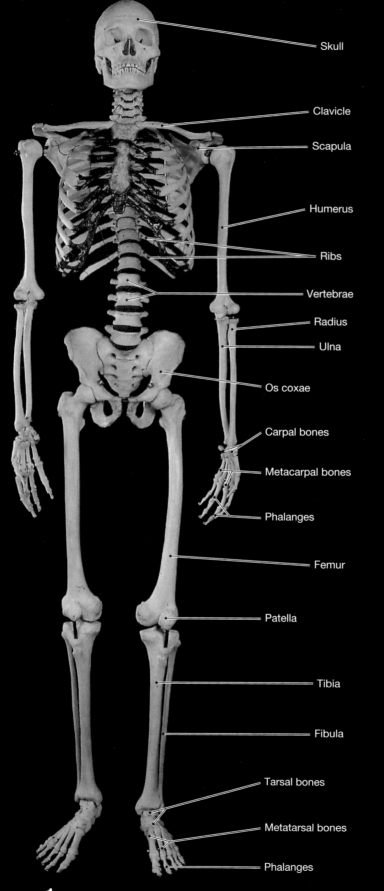

Skull

Clavicle

Scapula

Humerus

Ribs

Vertebrae

Radius

Ulna

Os coxae

Carpal bones

Metacarpal bones

Phalanges

Femur

Patella

Tibia

Fibula

Tarsal bones

Metatarsal bones

Phalanges

PLATE **1a** THE SKELETON, ANTERIOR VIEW

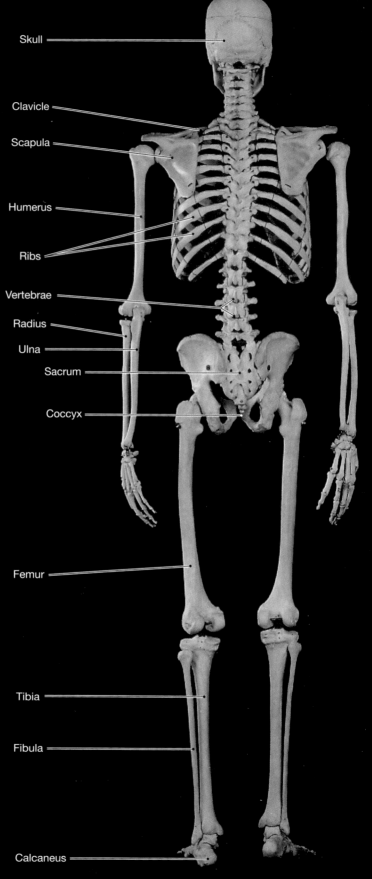

Skull

Clavicle

Scapula

Humerus

Ribs

Vertebrae

Radius

Ulna

Sacrum

Coccyx

Femur

Tibia

Fibula

Calcaneus

PLATE **1b** THE SKELETON, POSTERIOR VIEW

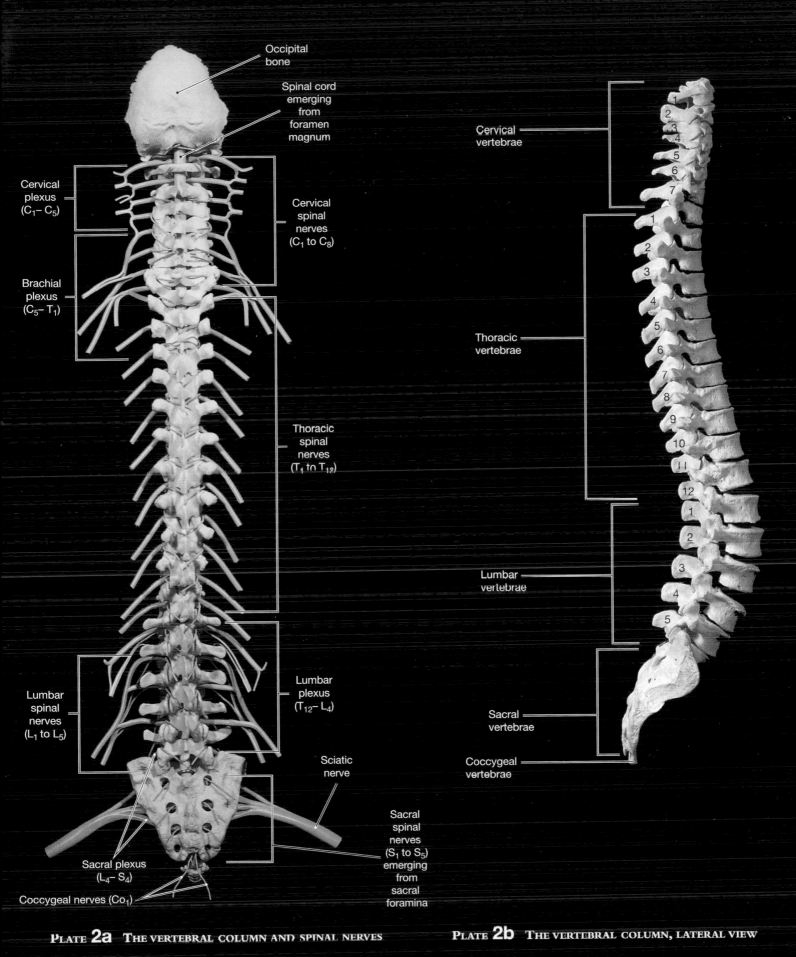

Occipital bone

Spinal cord emerging from foramen magnum

Cervical plexus (C_1– C_5)

Brachial plexus (C_5– T_1)

Cervical spinal nerves (C_1 to C_8)

Thoracic spinal nerves (T_1 to T_{12})

Lumbar spinal nerves (L_1 to L_5)

Lumbar plexus (T_{12}– L_4)

Sciatic nerve

Sacral plexus (L_4– S_4)

Coccygeal nerves (Co_1)

Sacral spinal nerves (S_1 to S_5) emerging from sacral foramina

Cervical vertebrae

Thoracic vertebrae

Lumbar vertebrae

Sacral vertebrae

Coccygeal vertebrae

PLATE 2a THE VERTEBRAL COLUMN AND SPINAL NERVES

PLATE 2b THE VERTEBRAL COLUMN, LATERAL VIEW

PLATE **3a** SURFACE ANATOMY OF THE
HEAD AND NECK, ANTERIOR VIEW

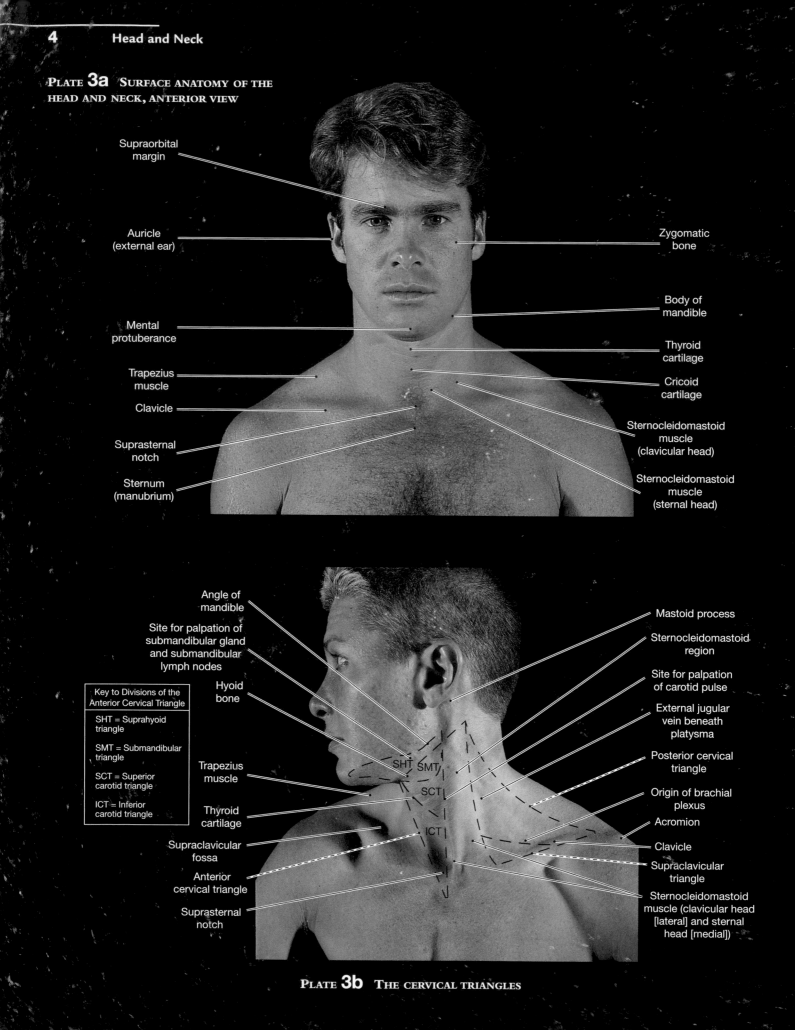

Supraorbital
margin

Auricle
(external ear)

Zygomatic
bone

Body of
mandible

Mental
protuberance

Thyroid
cartilage

Trapezius
muscle

Cricoid
cartilage

Clavicle

Sternocleidomastoid
muscle
(clavicular head)

Suprasternal
notch

Sternum
(manubrium)

Sternocleidomastoid
muscle
(sternal head)

Angle of
mandible

Mastoid process

Site for palpation of
submandibular gland
and submandibular
lymph nodes

Sternocleidomastoid
region

Site for palpation
of carotid pulse

Hyoid
bone

External jugular
vein beneath
platysma

Key to Divisions of the
Anterior Cervical Triangle

SHT = Suprahyoid
triangle

SMT = Submandibular
triangle

SCT = Superior
carotid triangle

ICT = Inferior
carotid triangle

Posterior cervical
triangle

Origin of brachial
plexus

Trapezius
muscle

Acromion

Thyroid
cartilage

Clavicle

Supraclavicular
fossa

Supraclavicular
triangle

Anterior
cervical triangle

Sternocleidomastoid
muscle (clavicular head
[lateral] and sternal
head [medial])

Suprasternal
notch

SHT   SMT

SCT

ICT

PLATE **3b** THE CERVICAL TRIANGLES

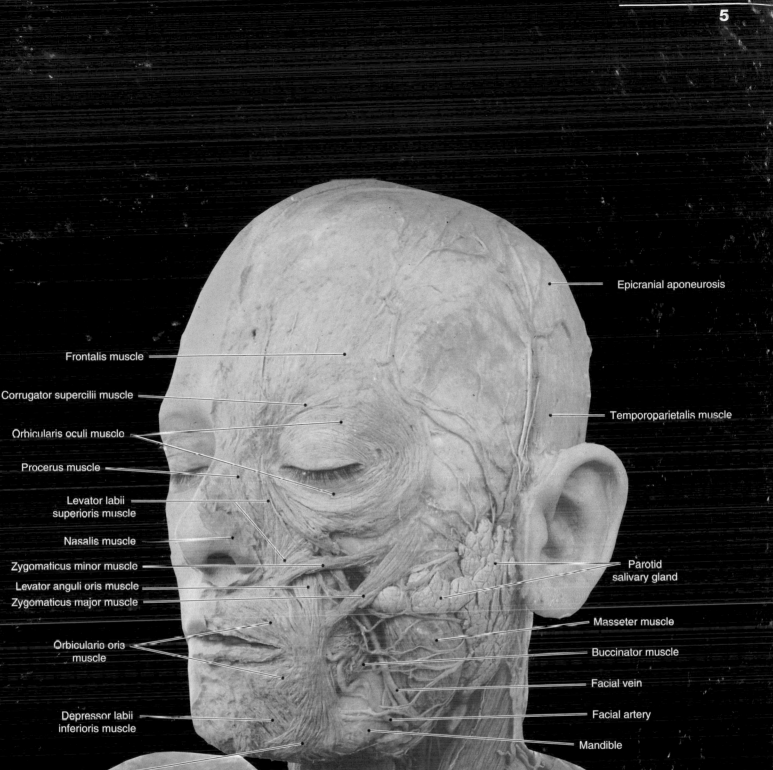

Epicranial aponeurosis

Frontalis muscle

Corrugator supercilii muscle

Temporoparietalis muscle

Orbicularis oculi muscle

Procerus muscle

Levator labii
superioris muscle

Nasalis muscle

Parotid
salivary gland

Zygomaticus minor muscle

Levator anguli oris muscle

Zygomaticus major muscle

Masseter muscle

Orbicularis oris
muscle

Buccinator muscle

Facial vein

Depressor labii
inferioris muscle

Facial artery

Mandible

Depressor anguli
oris muscle

Sternocleidomastoid
muscle

PLATE 3C SUPERFICIAL DISSECTION OF THE FACE, ANTEROLATERAL VIEW

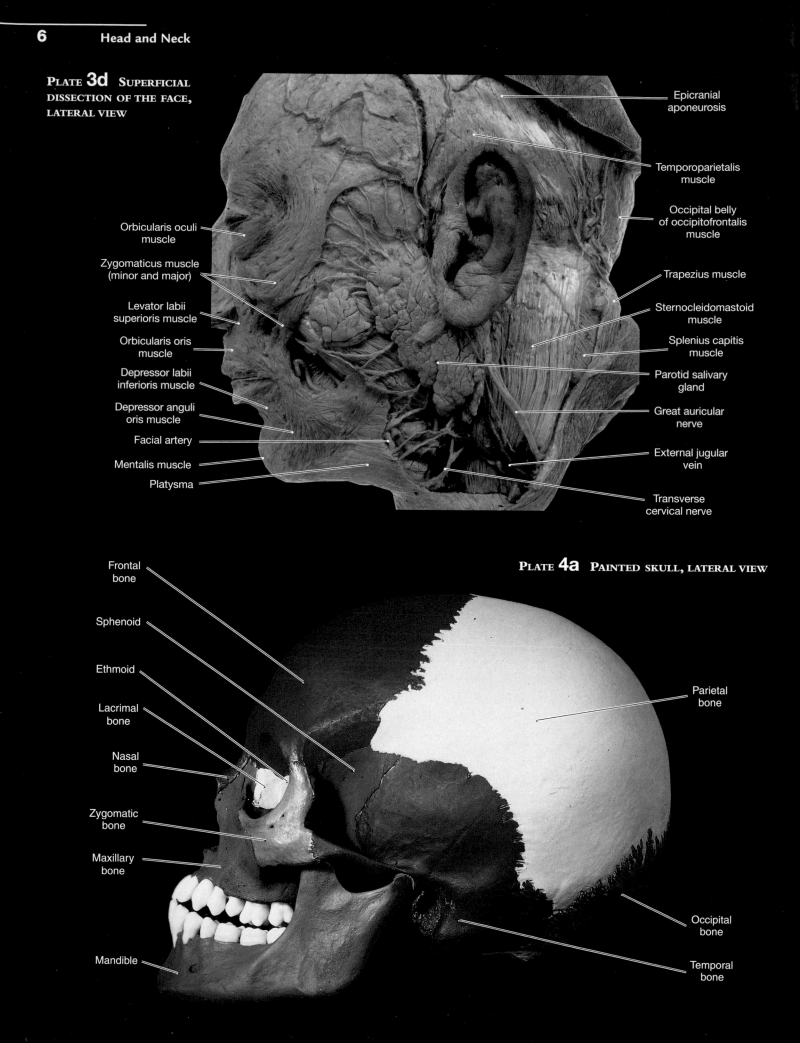

PLATE 3d SUPERFICIAL DISSECTION OF THE FACE, LATERAL VIEW

Epicranial aponeurosis

Temporoparietalis muscle

Occipital belly of occipitofrontalis muscle

Trapezius muscle

Sternocleidomastoid muscle

Splenius capitis muscle

Parotid salivary gland

Great auricular nerve

External jugular vein

Transverse cervical nerve

Orbicularis oculi muscle

Zygomaticus muscle (minor and major)

Levator labii superioris muscle

Orbicularis oris muscle

Depressor labii inferioris muscle

Depressor anguli oris muscle

Facial artery

Mentalis muscle

Platysma

PLATE 4a PAINTED SKULL, LATERAL VIEW

Frontal bone

Sphenoid

Ethmoid

Lacrimal bone

Nasal bone

Zygomatic bone

Maxillary bone

Mandible

Parietal bone

Occipital bone

Temporal bone

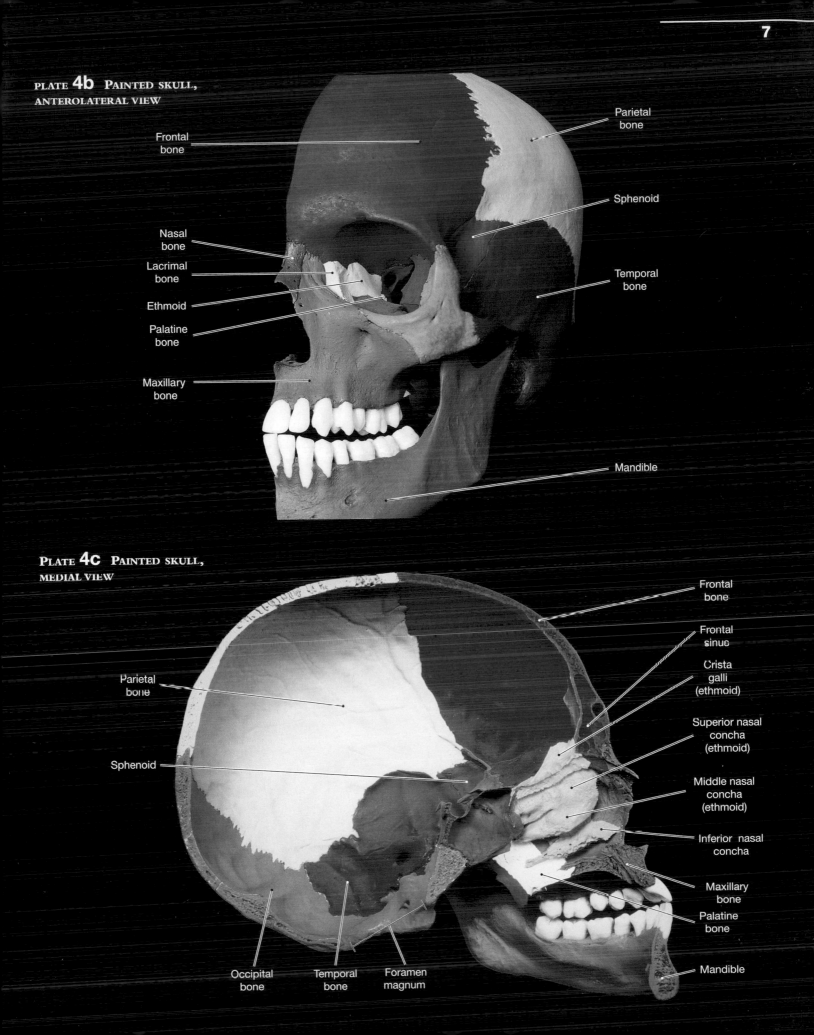

PLATE **4b** PAINTED SKULL, ANTEROLATERAL VIEW

Frontal bone

Parietal bone

Sphenoid

Nasal bone

Lacrimal bone

Ethmoid

Palatine bone

Temporal bone

Maxillary bone

Mandible

PLATE **4c** PAINTED SKULL, MEDIAL VIEW

Frontal bone

Frontal sinus

Crista galli (ethmoid)

Superior nasal concha (ethmoid)

Middle nasal concha (ethmoid)

Parietal bone

Sphenoid

Inferior nasal concha

Maxillary bone

Palatine bone

Occipital bone

Temporal bone

Foramen magnum

Mandible

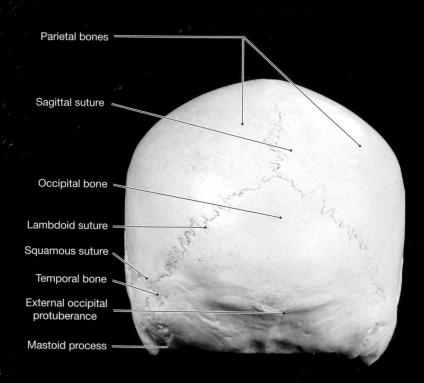

Parietal bones

Sagittal suture

Occipital bone

Lambdoid suture

Squamous suture

Temporal bone

External occipital protuberance

Mastoid process

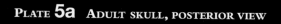

PLATE **5a** ADULT SKULL, POSTERIOR VIEW

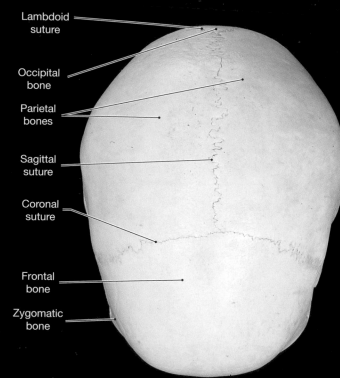

Lambdoid suture

Occipital bone

Parietal bones

Sagittal suture

Coronal suture

Frontal bone

Zygomatic bone

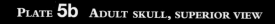

PLATE **5b** ADULT SKULL, SUPERIOR VIEW

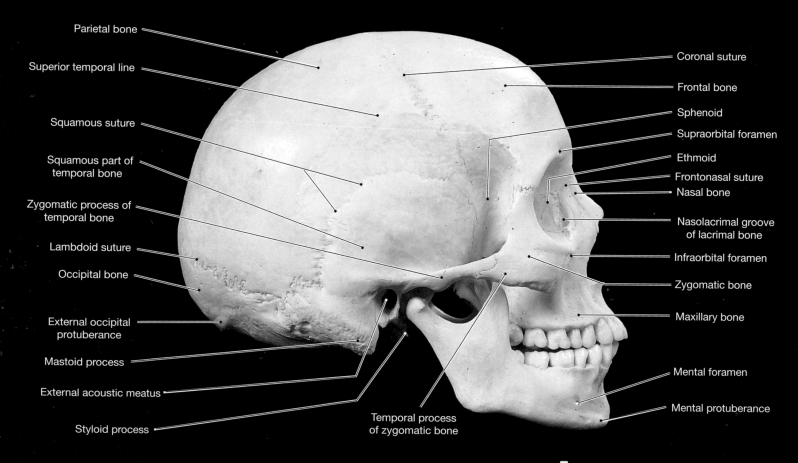

Parietal bone

Superior temporal line

Squamous suture

Squamous part of temporal bone

Zygomatic process of temporal bone

Lambdoid suture

Occipital bone

External occipital protuberance

Mastoid process

External acoustic meatus

Styloid process

Temporal process of zygomatic bone

Coronal suture

Frontal bone

Sphenoid

Supraorbital foramen

Ethmoid

Frontonasal suture

Nasal bone

Nasolacrimal groove of lacrimal bone

Infraorbital foramen

Zygomatic bone

Maxillary bone

Mental foramen

Mental protuberance

PLATE **5c** ADULT SKULL, LATERAL VIEW

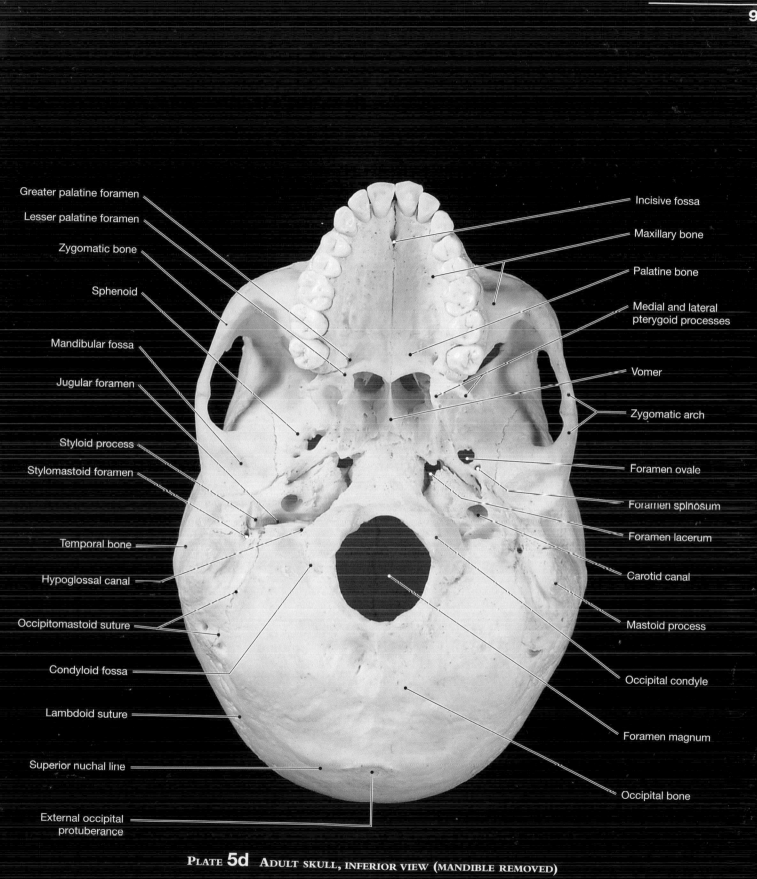

Greater palatine foramen

Lesser palatine foramen

Zygomatic bone

Sphenoid

Mandibular fossa

Jugular foramen

Styloid process

Stylomastoid foramen

Temporal bone

Hypoglossal canal

Occipitomastoid suture

Condyloid fossa

Lambdoid suture

Superior nuchal line

External occipital
protuberance

Incisive fossa

Maxillary bone

Palatine bone

Medial and lateral
pterygoid processes

Vomer

Zygomatic arch

Foramen ovale

Foramen spinosum

Foramen lacerum

Carotid canal

Mastoid process

Occipital condyle

Foramen magnum

Occipital bone

PLATE **5d** ADULT SKULL, INFERIOR VIEW (MANDIBLE REMOVED)

PLATE **5e** ADULT SKULL, ANTERIOR VIEW

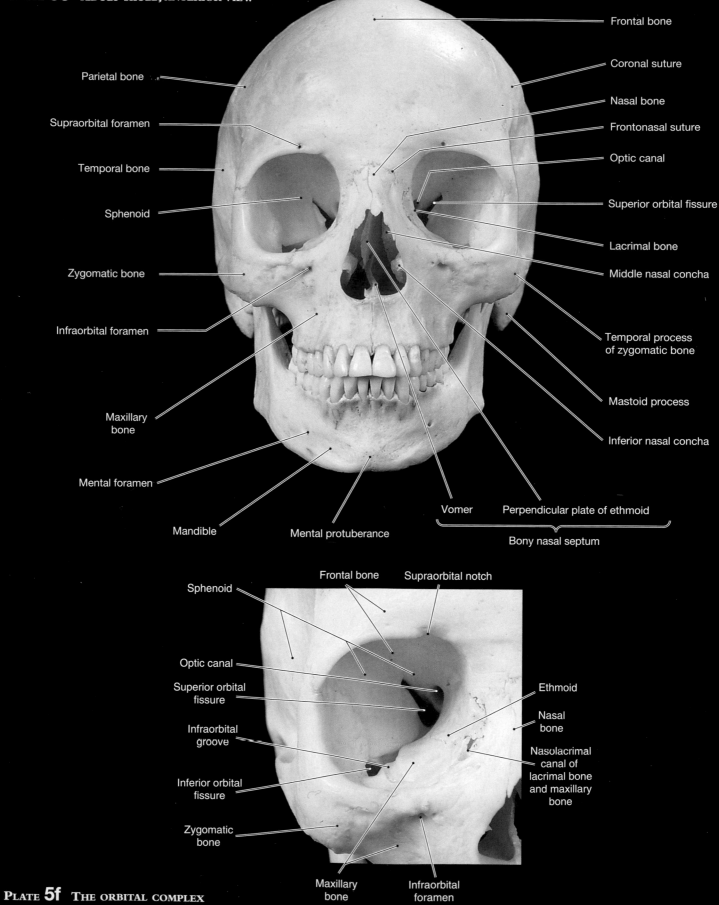

Frontal bone

Coronal suture

Nasal bone

Frontonasal suture

Optic canal

Superior orbital fissure

Lacrimal bone

Middle nasal concha

Temporal process of zygomatic bone

Mastoid process

Inferior nasal concha

Parietal bone

Supraorbital foramen

Temporal bone

Sphenoid

Zygomatic bone

Infraorbital foramen

Maxillary bone

Mental foramen

Mandible

Mental protuberance

Vomer

Perpendicular plate of ethmoid

Bony nasal septum

Frontal bone

Supraorbital notch

Sphenoid

Optic canal

Superior orbital fissure

Infraorbital groove

Inferior orbital fissure

Zygomatic bone

Ethmoid

Nasal bone

Nasolacrimal canal of lacrimal bone and maxillary bone

Maxillary bone

Infraorbital foramen

PLATE **5f** THE ORBITAL COMPLEX

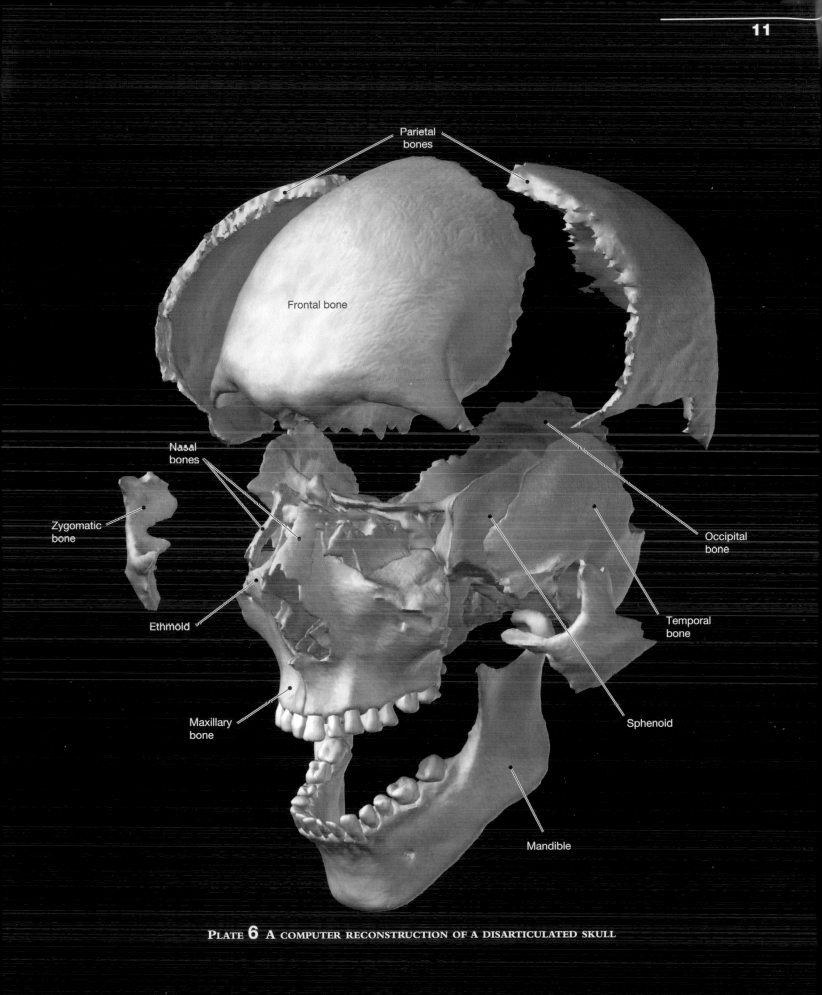

Parietal
bones

Frontal bone

Nasal
bones

Zygomatic
bone

Occipital
bone

Ethmoid

Temporal
bone

Maxillary
bone

Sphenoid

Mandible

PLATE 6 A COMPUTER RECONSTRUCTION OF A DISARTICULATED SKULL

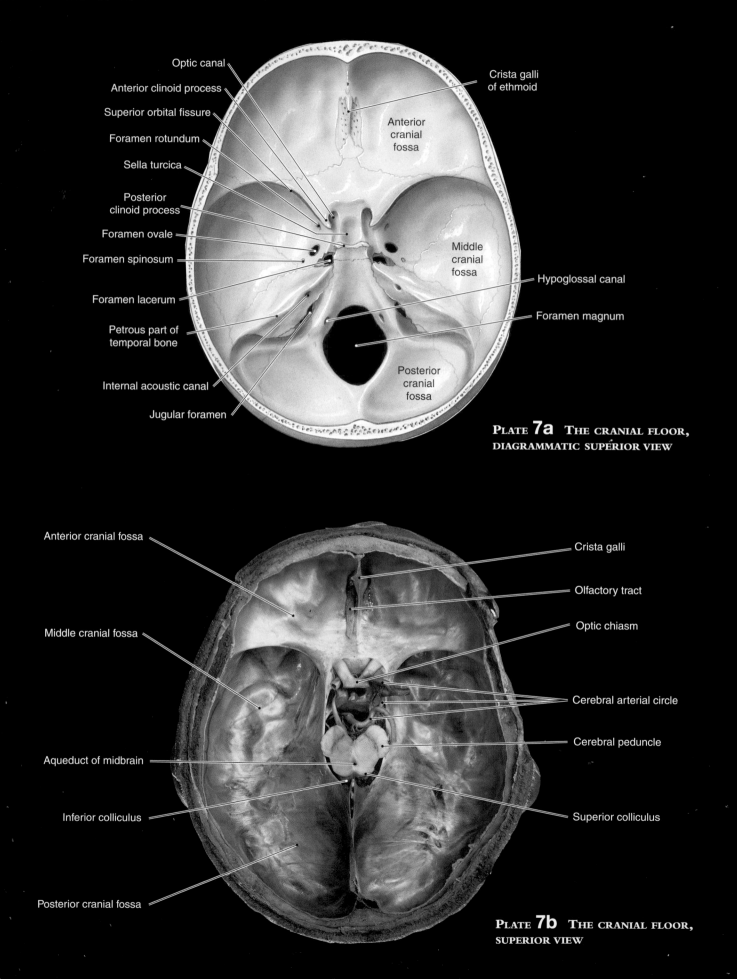

Optic canal
Anterior clinoid process
Superior orbital fissure
Foramen rotundum
Sella turcica
Posterior clinoid process
Foramen ovale
Foramen spinosum
Foramen lacerum
Petrous part of temporal bone
Internal acoustic canal
Jugular foramen

Crista galli of ethmoid
Anterior cranial fossa
Middle cranial fossa
Hypoglossal canal
Foramen magnum
Posterior cranial fossa

PLATE 7a THE CRANIAL FLOOR, DIAGRAMMATIC SUPERIOR VIEW

Anterior cranial fossa
Middle cranial fossa
Aqueduct of midbrain
Inferior colliculus
Posterior cranial fossa

Crista galli
Olfactory tract
Optic chiasm
Cerebral arterial circle
Cerebral peduncle
Superior colliculus

PLATE 7b THE CRANIAL FLOOR, SUPERIOR VIEW

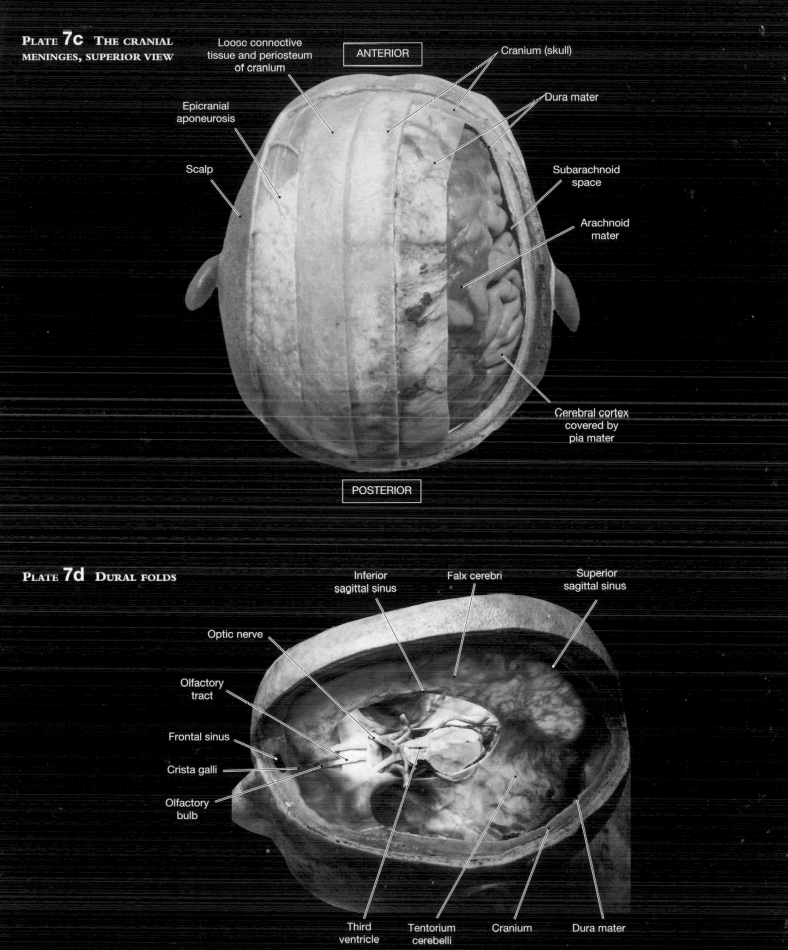

PLATE 7c THE CRANIAL MENINGES, SUPERIOR VIEW

Loose connective tissue and periosteum of cranium

Epicranial aponeurosis

Scalp

ANTERIOR

Cranium (skull)

Dura mater

Subarachnoid space

Arachnoid mater

Cerebral cortex covered by pia mater

POSTERIOR

PLATE 7d DURAL FOLDS

Inferior sagittal sinus

Falx cerebri

Superior sagittal sinus

Optic nerve

Olfactory tract

Frontal sinus

Crista galli

Olfactory bulb

Third ventricle

Tentorium cerebelli

Cranium

Dura mater

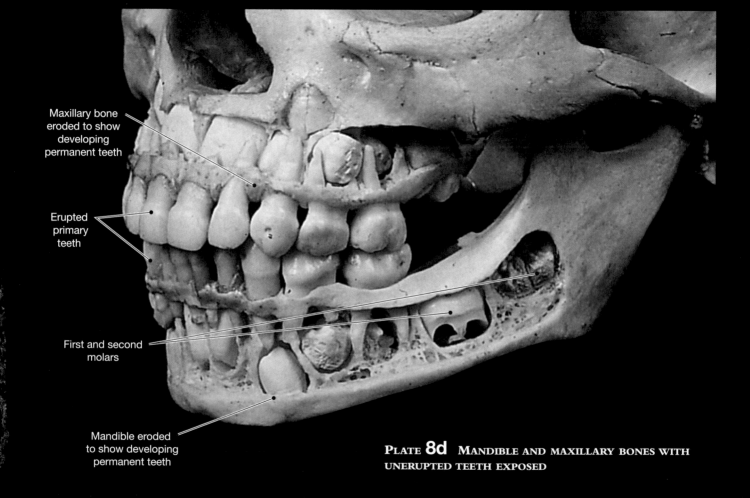

Maxillary bone
eroded to show
developing
permanent teeth

Erupted
primary
teeth

First and second
molars

Mandible eroded
to show developing
permanent teeth

PLATE 8d MANDIBLE AND MAXILLARY BONES WITH
UNERUPTED TEETH EXPOSED

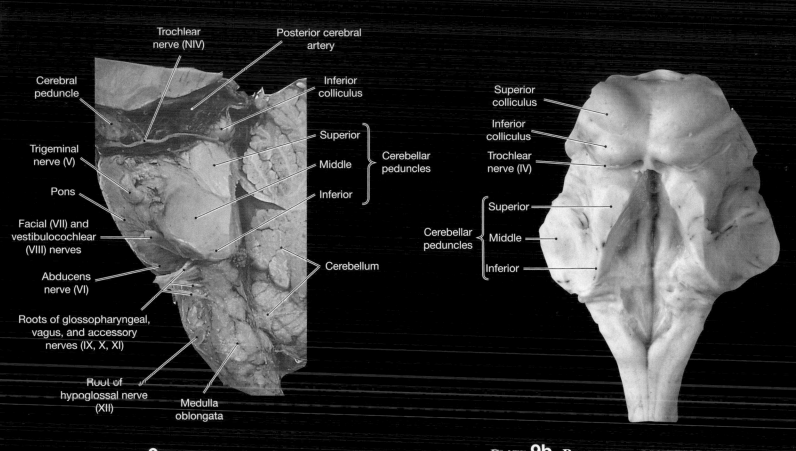

Trochlear nerve (NIV)

Posterior cerebral artery

Cerebral peduncle

Inferior colliculus

Trigeminal nerve (V)

Superior

Middle — Cerebellar peduncles

Pons

Inferior

Facial (VII) and vestibulocochlear (VIII) nerves

Abducens nerve (VI)

Cerebellum

Roots of glossopharyngeal, vagus, and accessory nerves (IX, X, XI)

Root of hypoglossal nerve (XII)

Medulla oblongata

PLATE **9a** BRAIN STEM, LATERAL VIEW

Superior colliculus

Inferior colliculus

Trochlear nerve (IV)

Superior

Cerebellar peduncles

Middle

Inferior

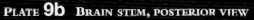

PLATE **9b** BRAIN STEM, POSTERIOR VIEW

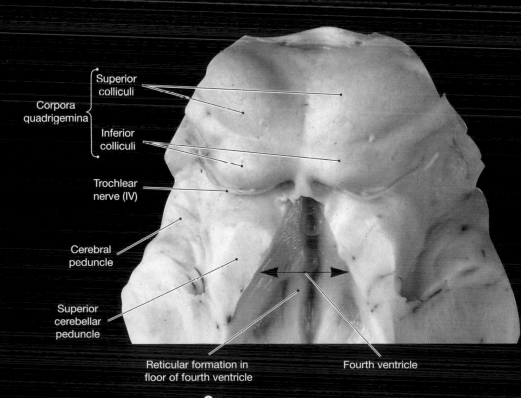

Superior colliculi

Corpora quadrigemina

Inferior colliculi

Trochlear nerve (IV)

Cerebral peduncle

Superior cerebellar peduncle

Reticular formation in floor of fourth ventricle

Fourth ventricle

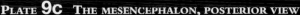

PLATE **9c** THE MESENCEPHALON, POSTERIOR VIEW

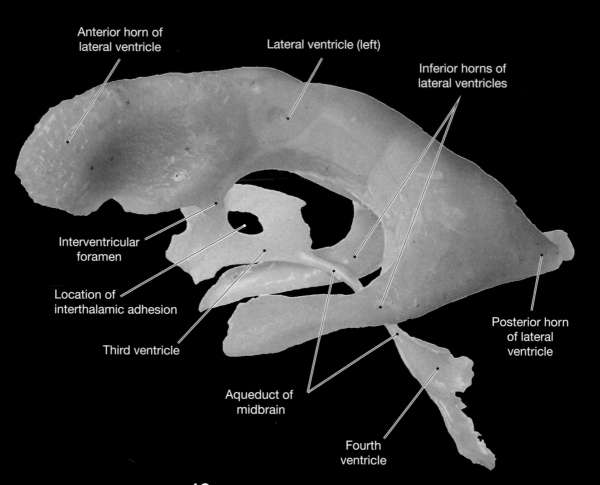

Anterior horn of
lateral ventricle

Lateral ventricle (left)

Inferior horns of
lateral ventricles

Interventricular
foramen

Location of
interthalamic adhesion

Third ventricle

Aqueduct of
midbrain

Fourth
ventricle

Posterior horn
of lateral
ventricle

PLATE **10**   VENTRICLE CASTING, LATERAL VIEW

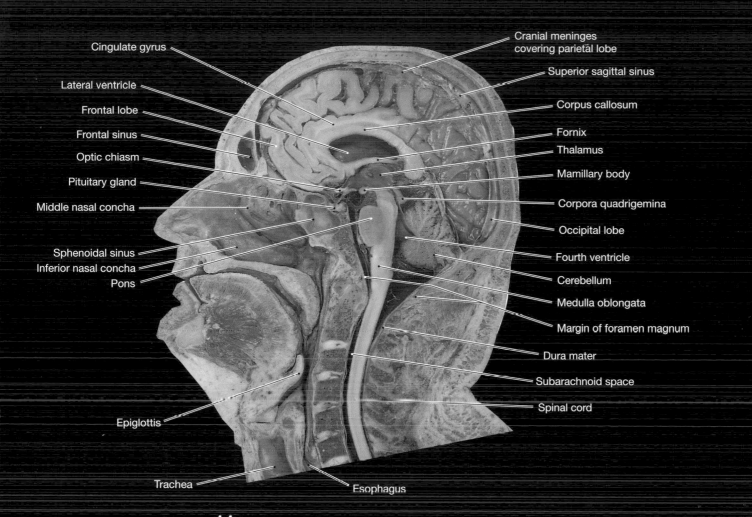

Cingulate gyrus

Lateral ventricle

Frontal lobe

Frontal sinus

Optic chiasm

Pituitary gland

Middle nasal concha

Sphenoidal sinus
Inferior nasal concha
Pons

Epiglottis

Trachea

Esophagus

Cranial meninges
covering parietal lobe

Superior sagittal sinus

Corpus callosum

Fornix

Thalamus

Mamillary body

Corpora quadrigemina

Occipital lobe

Fourth ventricle

Cerebellum

Medulla oblongata

Margin of foramen magnum

Dura mater

Subarachnoid space

Spinal cord

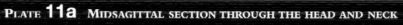

PLATE 11a MIDSAGITTAL SECTION THROUGH THE HEAD AND NECK

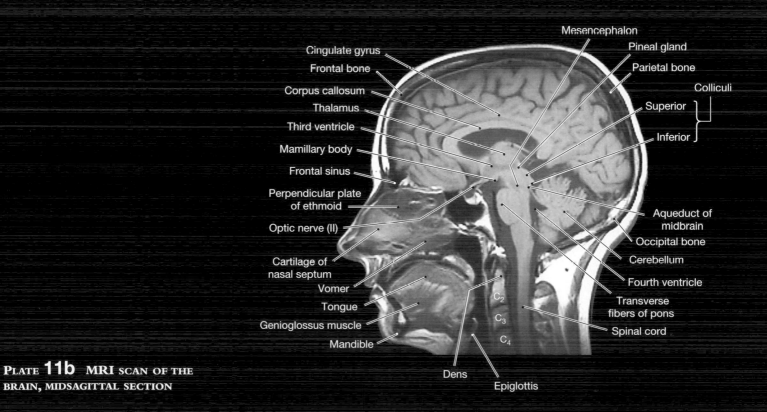

Cingulate gyrus

Frontal bone

Corpus callosum

Thalamus

Third ventricle

Mamillary body

Frontal sinus

Perpendicular plate
of ethmoid

Optic nerve (II)

Cartilage of
nasal septum

Vomer

Tongue

Genioglossus muscle

Mandible

Mesencephalon

Pineal gland

Parietal bone

Colliculi

Superior

Inferior

Aqueduct of
midbrain

Occipital bone

Cerebellum

Fourth ventricle

Transverse
fibers of pons

Spinal cord

C₂

C₃

C₄

Dens

Epiglottis

PLATE 11b MRI SCAN OF THE
BRAIN, MIDSAGITTAL SECTION

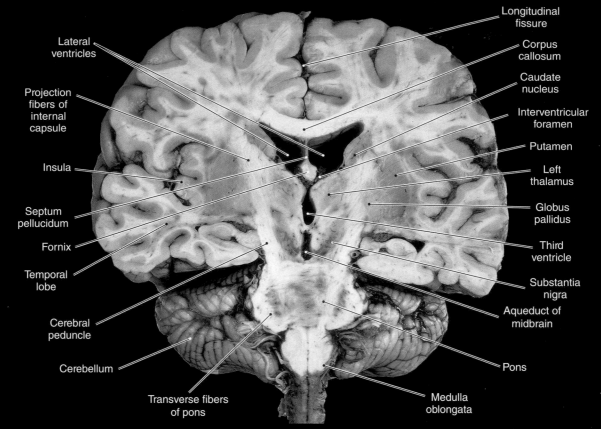

Lateral
ventricles

Projection
fibers of
internal
capsule

Insula

Septum
pellucidum

Fornix

Temporal
lobe

Cerebral
peduncle

Cerebellum

Transverse fibers
of pons

Longitudinal
fissure

Corpus
callosum

Caudate
nucleus

Interventricular
foramen

Putamen

Left
thalamus

Globus
pallidus

Third
ventricle

Substantia
nigra

Aqueduct of
midbrain

Pons

Medulla
oblongata

PLATE 11c CORONAL SECTION THROUGH THE BRAIN AT THE LEVEL OF THE MESENCEPHALON AND PONS

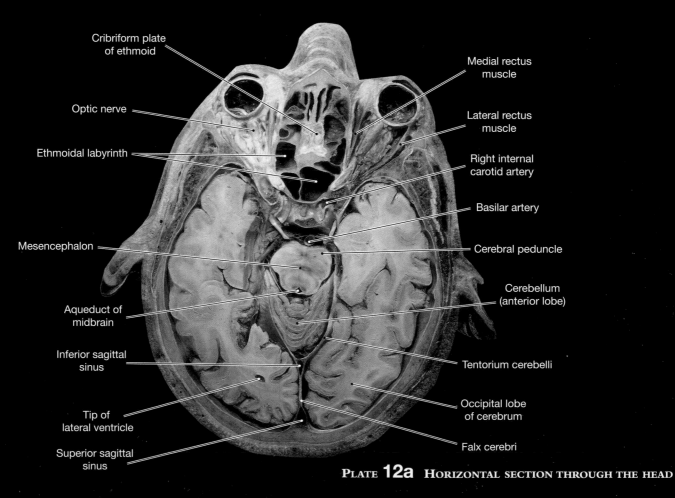

Cribriform plate
of ethmoid

Optic nerve

Ethmoidal labyrinth

Mesencephalon

Aqueduct of
midbrain

Inferior sagittal
sinus

Tip of
lateral ventricle

Superior sagittal
sinus

Medial rectus
muscle

Lateral rectus
muscle

Right internal
carotid artery

Basilar artery

Cerebral peduncle

Cerebellum
(anterior lobe)

Tentorium cerebelli

Occipital lobe
of cerebrum

Falx cerebri

PLATE 12a HORIZONTAL SECTION THROUGH THE HEAD

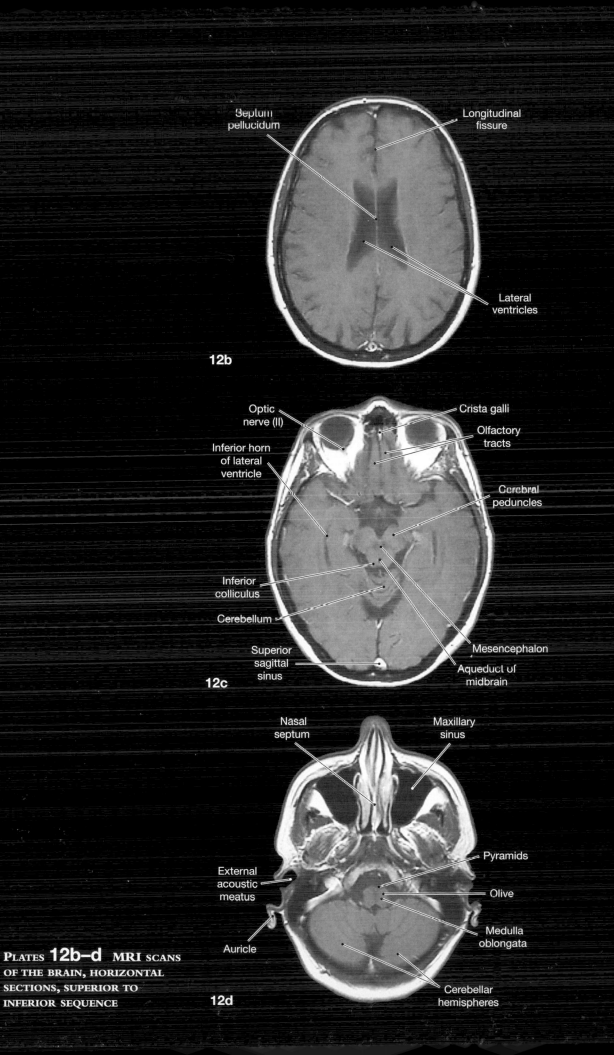

12b

- Septum pellucidum
- Longitudinal fissure
- Lateral ventricles

12c

- Optic nerve (II)
- Crista galli
- Olfactory tracts
- Inferior horn of lateral ventricle
- Cerebral peduncles
- Inferior colliculus
- Cerebellum
- Superior sagittal sinus
- Mesencephalon
- Aqueduct of midbrain

12d

- Nasal septum
- Maxillary sinus
- Pyramids
- External acoustic meatus
- Olive
- Medulla oblongata
- Auricle
- Cerebellar hemispheres

PLATES **12b–d** MRI SCANS OF THE BRAIN, HORIZONTAL SECTIONS, SUPERIOR TO INFERIOR SEQUENCE

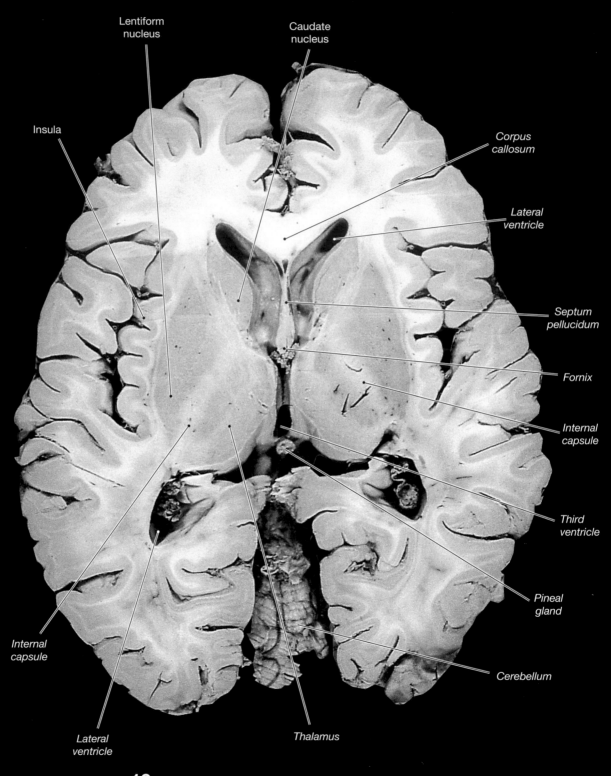

Lentiform
nucleus

Caudate
nucleus

Insula

*Corpus
callosum*

*Lateral
ventricle*

*Septum
pellucidum*

Fornix

*Internal
capsule*

*Third
ventricle*

*Pineal
gland*

Cerebellum

*Internal
capsule*

*Lateral
ventricle*

Thalamus

PLATE **13a**   A HORIZONTAL SECTION THROUGH THE BRAIN

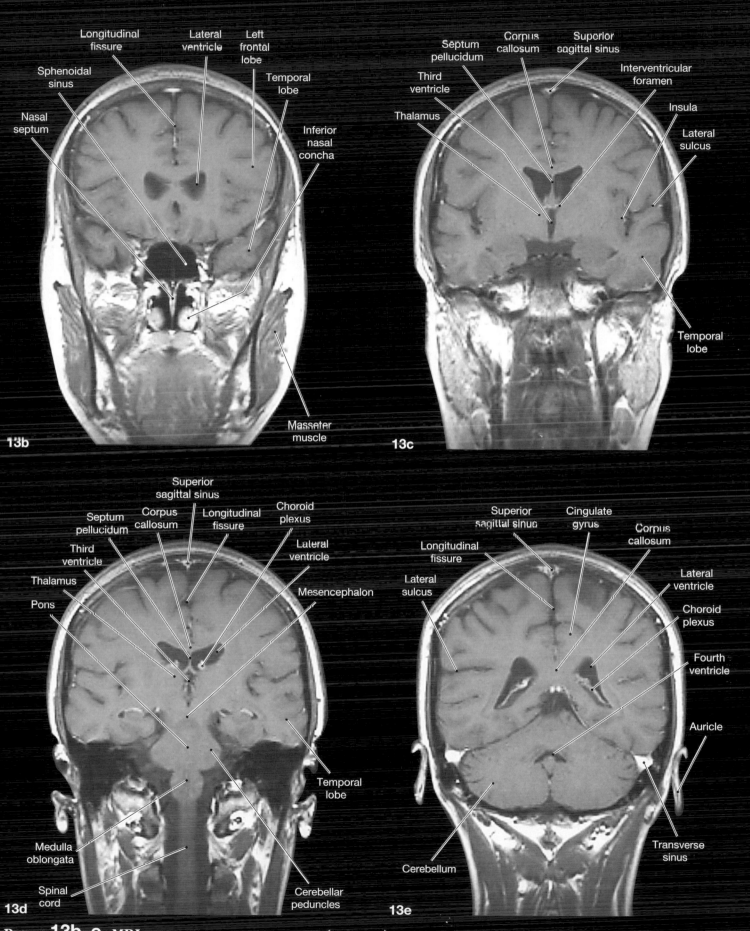

13b

Longitudinal fissure
Lateral ventricle
Left frontal lobe
Sphenoidal sinus
Temporal lobe
Nasal septum
Inferior nasal concha
Masseter muscle

13c

Septum pellucidum
Corpus callosum
Superior sagittal sinus
Third ventricle
Interventricular foramen
Thalamus
Insula
Lateral sulcus
Temporal lobe

13d

Superior sagittal sinus
Septum pellucidum
Corpus callosum
Longitudinal fissure
Choroid plexus
Third ventricle
Lateral ventricle
Thalamus
Mesencephalon
Pons
Temporal lobe
Medulla oblongata
Spinal cord
Cerebellar peduncles

13e

Superior sagittal sinus
Cingulate gyrus
Corpus callosum
Longitudinal fissure
Lateral sulcus
Lateral ventricle
Choroid plexus
Fourth ventricle
Auricle
Cerebellum
Transverse sinus

PLATES **13b–e** MRI SCANS OF THE BRAIN, FRONTAL (CORONAL) SECTIONS, ANTERIOR TO POSTERIOR SEQUENCE

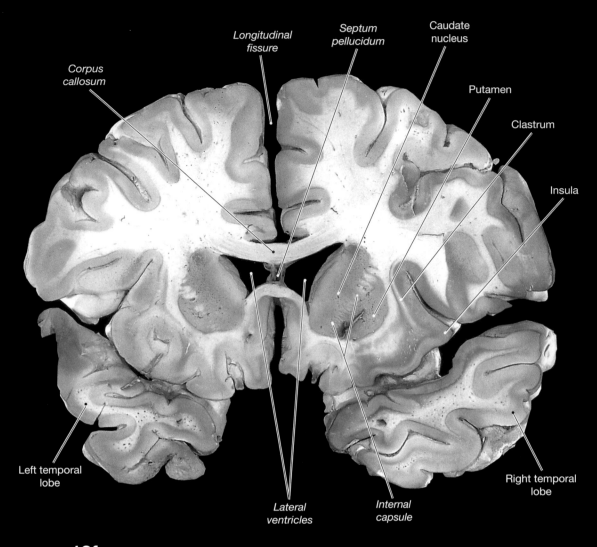

Corpus callosum

Longitudinal fissure

Septum pellucidum

Caudate nucleus

Putamen

Clastrum

Insula

Left temporal lobe

Right temporal lobe

Lateral ventricles

Internal capsule

PLATE **13f** FRONTAL SECTION THROUGH THE BRAIN AT THE LEVEL OF THE BASAL NUCLEI

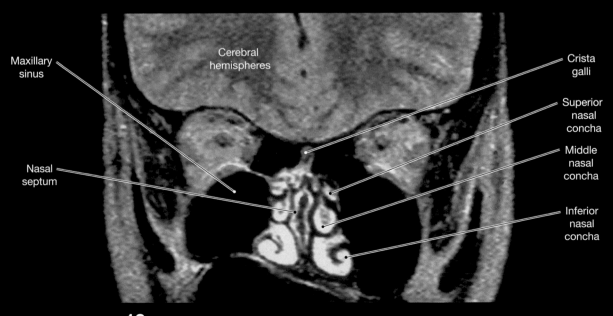

Maxillary sinus

Cerebral hemispheres

Crista galli

Superior nasal concha

Middle nasal concha

Nasal septum

Inferior nasal concha

PLATE **13g** MRI SCAN, CORONAL SECTION SHOWING PARANASAL SINUSES

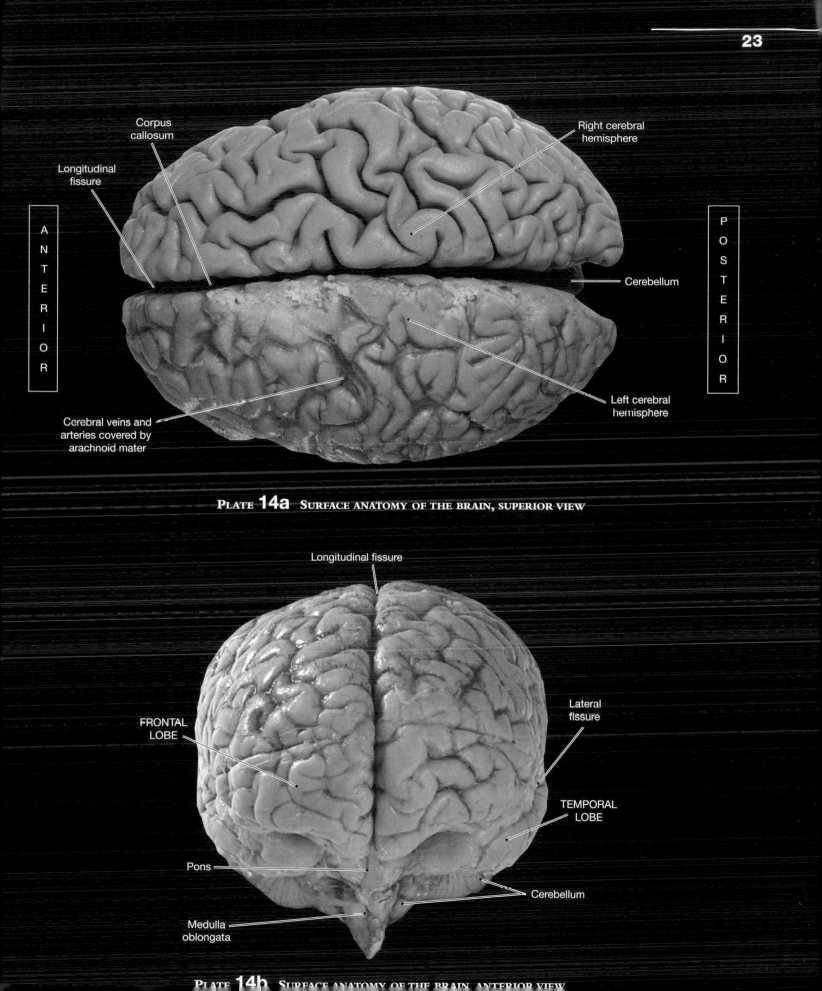

Corpus callosum

Longitudinal fissure

Right cerebral hemisphere

ANTERIOR

POSTERIOR

Cerebellum

Left cerebral hemisphere

Cerebral veins and arteries covered by arachnoid mater

PLATE **14a** SURFACE ANATOMY OF THE BRAIN, SUPERIOR VIEW

Longitudinal fissure

FRONTAL LOBE

Lateral fissure

TEMPORAL LOBE

Pons

Cerebellum

Medulla oblongata

PLATE **14b** SURFACE ANATOMY OF THE BRAIN, ANTERIOR VIEW

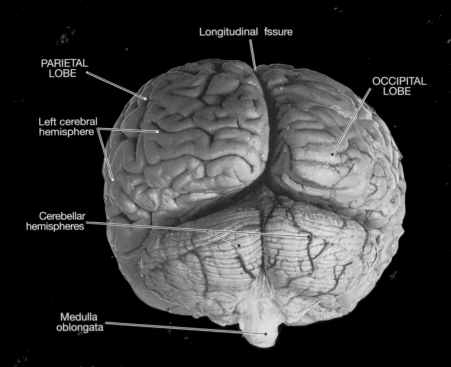

Longitudinal fissure

PARIETAL
LOBE

OCCIPITAL
LOBE

Left cerebral
hemisphere

Cerebellar
hemispheres

Medulla
oblongata

PLATE **14c** SURFACE ANATOMY OF THE BRAIN, POSTERIOR VIEW

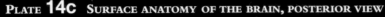

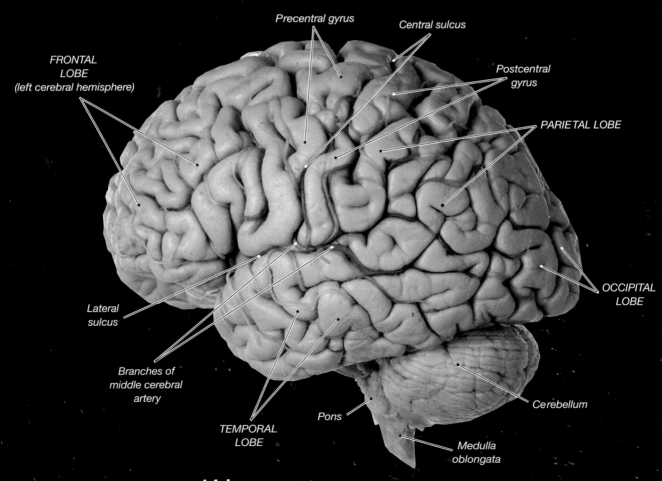

Precentral gyrus

Central sulcus

FRONTAL
LOBE
(left cerebral hemisphere)

Postcentral
gyrus

PARIETAL LOBE

OCCIPITAL
LOBE

Lateral
sulcus

Branches of
middle cerebral
artery

Cerebellum

Pons

TEMPORAL
LOBE

Medulla
oblongata

PLATE **14d** SURFACE ANATOMY OF THE BRAIN, LATERAL VIEW

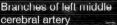

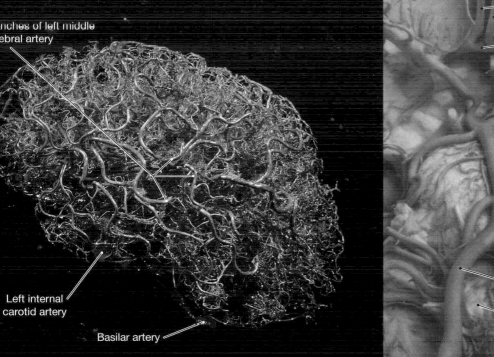

Branches of left middle cerebral artery

Left internal carotid artery

Basilar artery

PLATE 15a ARTERIAL CIRCULATION TO THE BRAIN, LATERAL VIEW OF CORROSION CAST

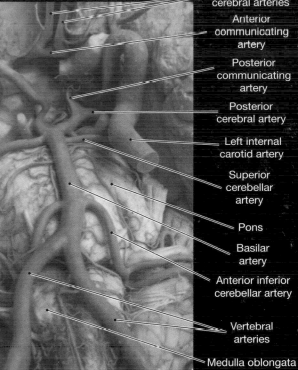

cerebral arteries

Anterior communicating artery

Posterior communicating artery

Posterior cerebral artery

Left internal carotid artery

Superior cerebellar artery

Pons

Basilar artery

Anterior inferior cerebellar artery

Vertebral arteries

Medulla oblongata

PLATE 15c ARTERIES ON THE INFERIOR SURFACE OF THE BRAIN

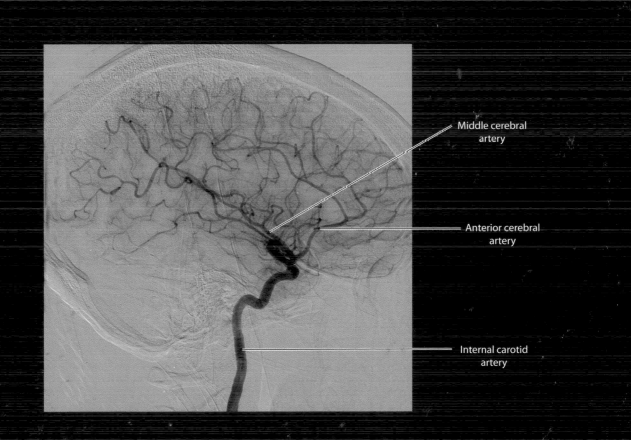

Middle cerebral artery

Anterior cerebral artery

Internal carotid artery

PLATE 15b CRANIAL ANGIOGRAM

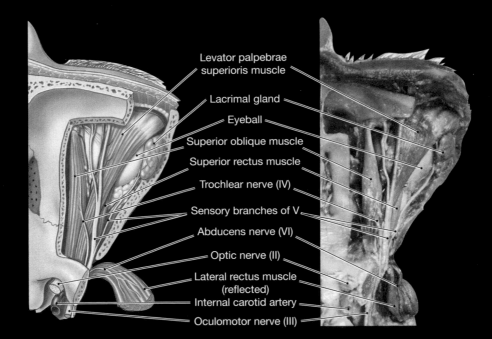

Levator palpebrae
superioris muscle

Lacrimal gland

Eyeball

Superior oblique muscle

Superior rectus muscle

Trochlear nerve (IV)

Sensory branches of V

Abducens nerve (VI)

Optic nerve (II)

Lateral rectus muscle
(reflected)

Internal carotid artery

Oculomotor nerve (III)

PLATES 16a–b   ACCESSORY STRUCTURES OF THE EYE, SUPERIOR VIEW

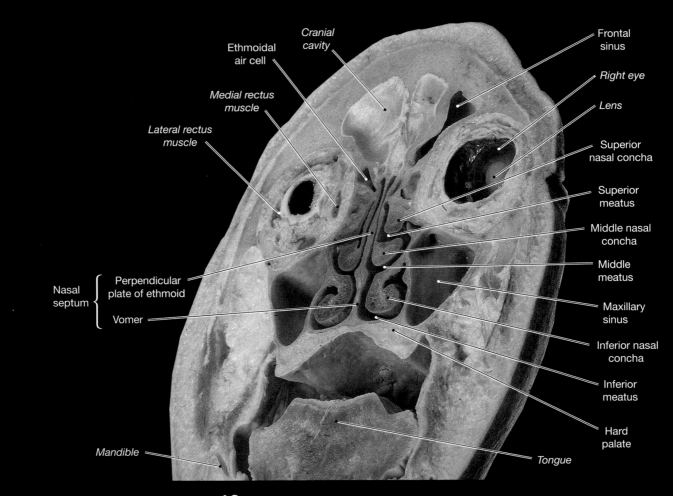

Ethmoidal
air cell

*Cranial
cavity*

Frontal
sinus

Medial rectus
muscle

Right eye

Lens

Lateral rectus
muscle

Superior
nasal concha

Superior
meatus

Middle nasal
concha

Middle
meatus

Nasal
septum {

Perpendicular
plate of ethmoid

Vomer

Maxillary
sinus

Inferior nasal
concha

Inferior
meatus

Mandible

Tongue

Hard
palate

PLATE 16c   FRONTAL SECTION THROUGH THE FACE

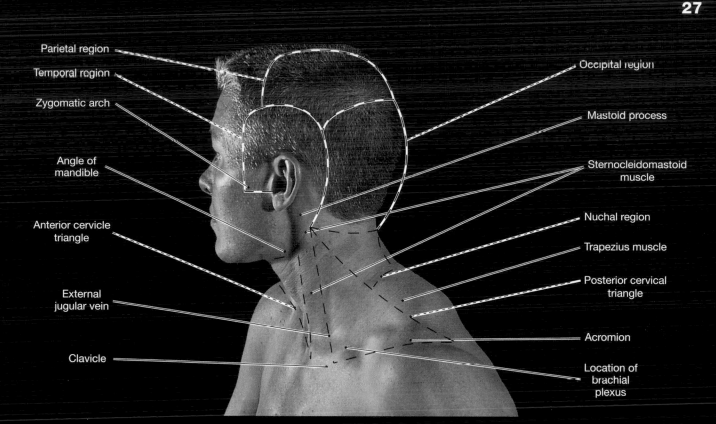

Parietal region

Temporal region

Zygomatic arch

Angle of mandible

Anterior cervicle triangle

External jugular vein

Clavicle

Occipital region

Mastoid process

Sternocleidomastoid muscle

Nuchal region

Trapezius muscle

Posterior cervical triangle

Acromion

Location of brachial plexus

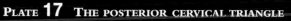

PLATE 17 THE POSTERIOR CERVICAL TRIANGLE

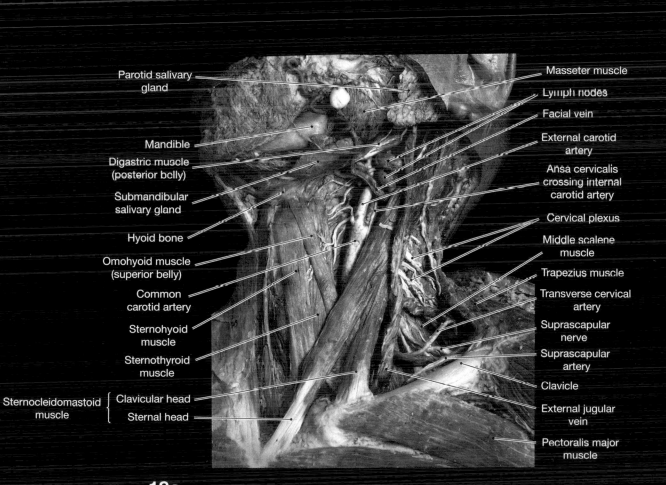

Parotid salivary gland

Mandible

Digastric muscle (posterior belly)

Submandibular salivary gland

Hyoid bone

Omohyoid muscle (superior belly)

Common carotid artery

Sternohyoid muscle

Sternothyroid muscle

Sternocleidomastoid muscle

Clavicular head

Sternal head

Masseter muscle

Lymph nodes

Facial vein

External carotid artery

Ansa cervicalis crossing internal carotid artery

Cervical plexus

Middle scalene muscle

Trapezius muscle

Transverse cervical artery

Suprascapular nerve

Suprascapular artery

Clavicle

External jugular vein

Pectoralis major muscle

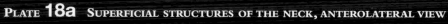

PLATE 18a SUPERFICIAL STRUCTURES OF THE NECK, ANTEROLATERAL VIEW

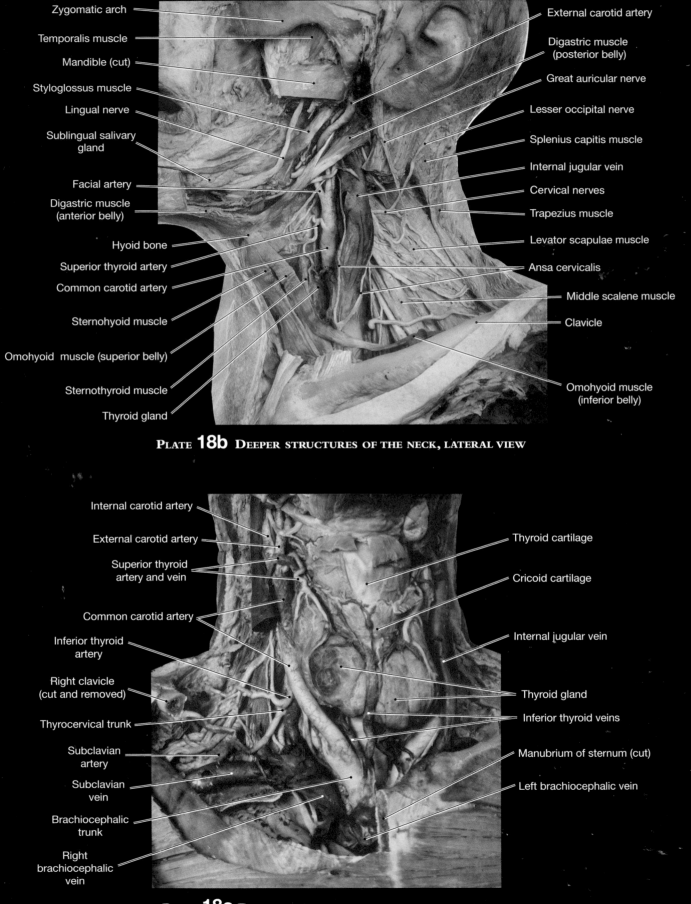

Zygomatic arch

Temporalis muscle

Mandible (cut)

Styloglossus muscle

Lingual nerve

Sublingual salivary gland

Facial artery

Digastric muscle (anterior belly)

Hyoid bone

Superior thyroid artery

Common carotid artery

Sternohyoid muscle

Omohyoid muscle (superior belly)

Sternothyroid muscle

Thyroid gland

External carotid artery

Digastric muscle (posterior belly)

Great auricular nerve

Lesser occipital nerve

Splenius capitis muscle

Internal jugular vein

Cervical nerves

Trapezius muscle

Levator scapulae muscle

Ansa cervicalis

Middle scalene muscle

Clavicle

Omohyoid muscle (inferior belly)

PLATE 18b DEEPER STRUCTURES OF THE NECK, LATERAL VIEW

Internal carotid artery

External carotid artery

Superior thyroid artery and vein

Common carotid artery

Inferior thyroid artery

Right clavicle (cut and removed)

Thyrocervical trunk

Subclavian artery

Subclavian vein

Brachiocephalic trunk

Right brachiocephalic vein

Thyroid cartilage

Cricoid cartilage

Internal jugular vein

Thyroid gland

Inferior thyroid veins

Manubrium of sternum (cut)

Left brachiocephalic vein

PLATE 18c DEEPER STRUCTURES OF THE NECK, ANTERIOR VIEW

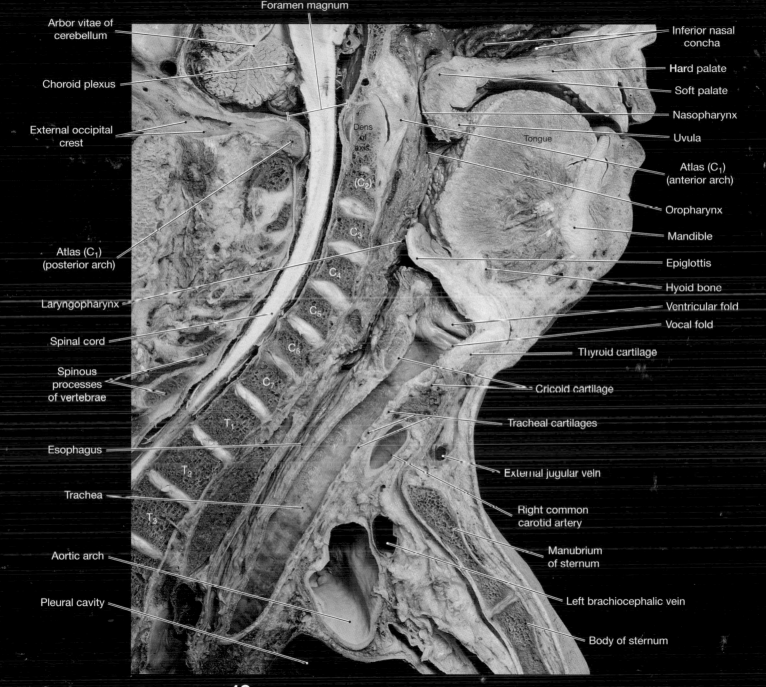

Foramen magnum

Arbor vitae of cerebellum

Choroid plexus

External occipital crest

Atlas (C₁) (posterior arch)

Laryngopharynx

Spinal cord

Spinous processes of vertebrae

Esophagus

Trachea

Aortic arch

Pleural cavity

Inferior nasal concha

Hard palate

Soft palate

Nasopharynx

Uvula

Atlas (C₁) (anterior arch)

Oropharynx

Mandible

Epiglottis

Hyoid bone

Ventricular fold

Vocal fold

Thyroid cartilage

Cricoid cartilage

Tracheal cartilages

External jugular vein

Right common carotid artery

Manubrium of sternum

Left brachiocephalic vein

Body of sternum

Dens of axis

(C₂)

C₃

C₄

C₅

C₆

C₇

T₁

T₂

T₃

Tongue

PLATE 19 MIDSAGITTAL SECTION THROUGH THE HEAD AND NECK

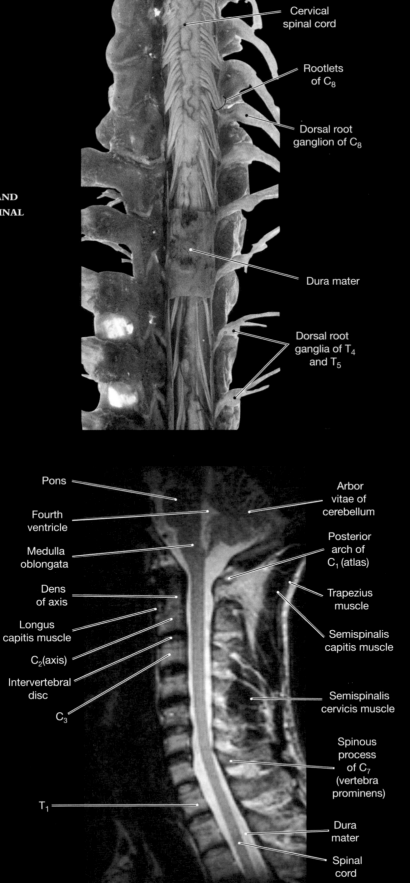

Cervical
spinal cord

Rootlets
of C_8

Dorsal root
ganglion of C_8

PLATE 20a THE CERVICAL AND
THORACIC REGIONS OF THE SPINAL
CORD, POSTERIOR VIEW

Dura mater

Dorsal root
ganglia of T_4
and T_5

Pons

Fourth
ventricle

Medulla
oblongata

Dens
of axis

Longus
capitis muscle

C_2(axis)

Intervertebral
disc

C_3

T_1

Arbor
vitae of
cerebellum

Posterior
arch of
C_1 (atlas)

Trapezius
muscle

Semispinalis
capitis muscle

Semispinalis
cervicis muscle

Spinous
process
of C_7
(vertebra
prominens)

Dura
mater

Spinal
cord

PLATE 20b MRI SCAN OF CERVICAL REGION, SAGITTAL SECTION

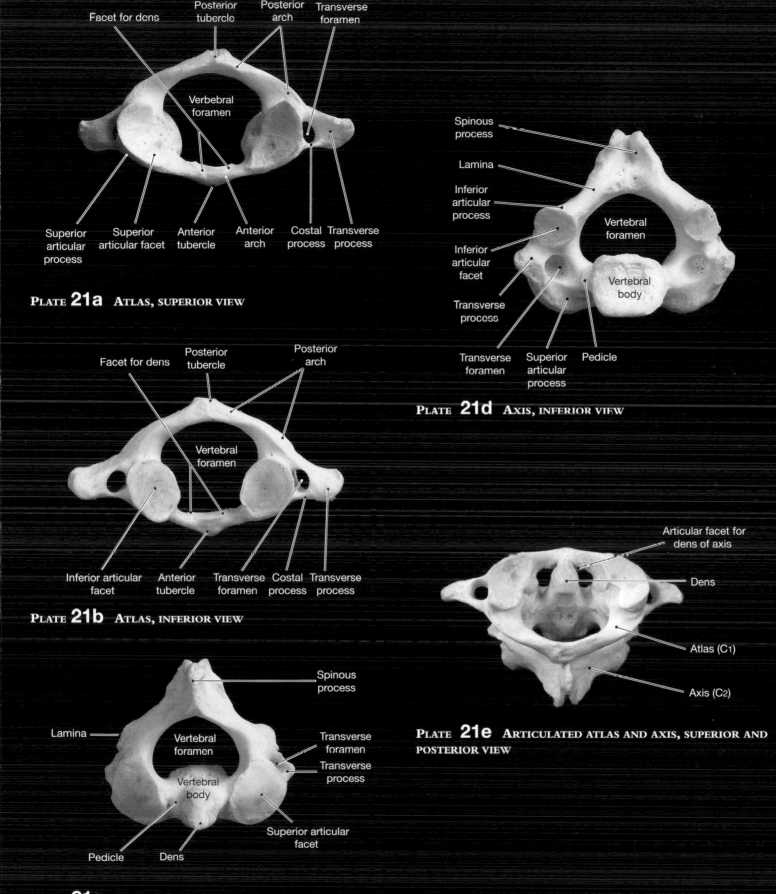

Facet for dens Posterior tubercle Posterior arch Transverse foramen

Verbebral foramen

Superior articular process Superior articular facet Anterior tubercle Anterior arch Costal process Transverse process

PLATE 21a ATLAS, SUPERIOR VIEW

Facet for dens Posterior tubercle Posterior arch

Vertebral foramen

Inferior articular facet Anterior tubercle Transverse foramen Costal process Transverse process

PLATE 21b ATLAS, INFERIOR VIEW

Spinous process

Lamina

Vertebral foramen

Vertebral body

Pedicle Dens Superior articular facet

PLATE 21c AXIS, SUPERIOR VIEW

Spinous process

Lamina

Inferior articular process

Inferior articular facet

Transverse process

Vertebral foramen

Vertebral body

Transverse foramen Superior articular process Pedicle

PLATE 21d AXIS, INFERIOR VIEW

Articular facet for dens of axis

Dens

Atlas (C1)

Axis (C2)

PLATE 21e ARTICULATED ATLAS AND AXIS, SUPERIOR AND POSTERIOR VIEW

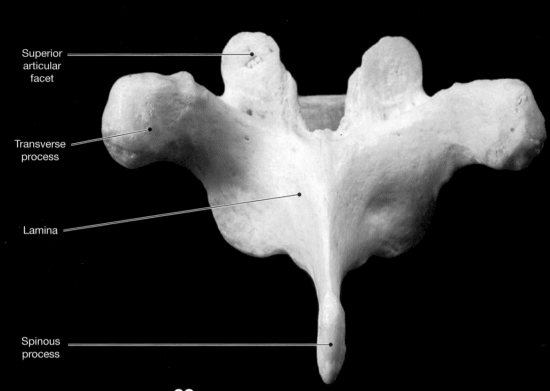

Superior
articular
facet

Transverse
process

Lamina

Spinous
process

PLATE **22a** THORACIC VERTEBRA, POSTERIOR VIEW

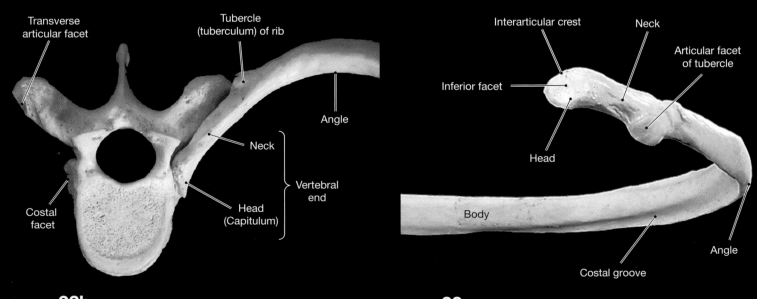

Transverse
articular facet

Tubercle
(tuberculum) of rib

Angle

Neck

Vertebral
end

Head
(Capitulum)

Costal
facet

PLATE **22b** THORACIC VERTEBRA AND RIB, SUPERIOR VIEW

Interarticular crest

Neck

Articular facet
of tubercle

Inferior facet

Head

Body

Angle

Costal groove

PLATE **22c** REPRESENTATIVE RIB, POSTERIOR VIEW

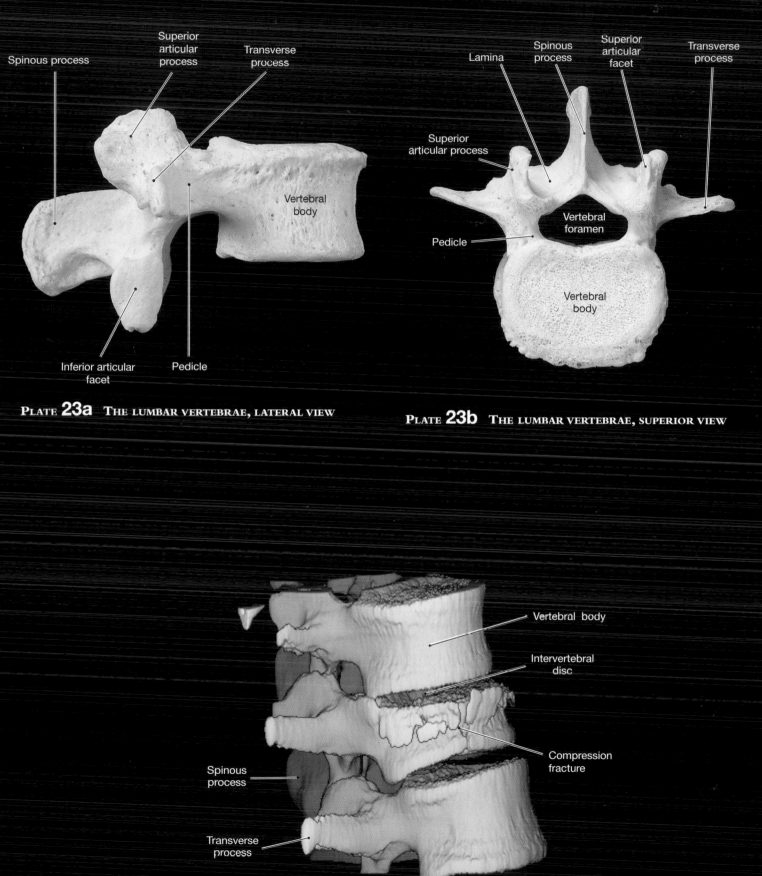

Spinous process

Superior articular process

Transverse process

Vertebral body

Inferior articular facet

Pedicle

PLATE 23a THE LUMBAR VERTEBRAE, LATERAL VIEW

Lamina

Spinous process

Superior articular facet

Transverse process

Superior articular process

Vertebral foramen

Pedicle

Vertebral body

PLATE 23b THE LUMBAR VERTEBRAE, SUPERIOR VIEW

Vertebral body

Intervertebral disc

Compression fracture

Spinous process

Transverse process

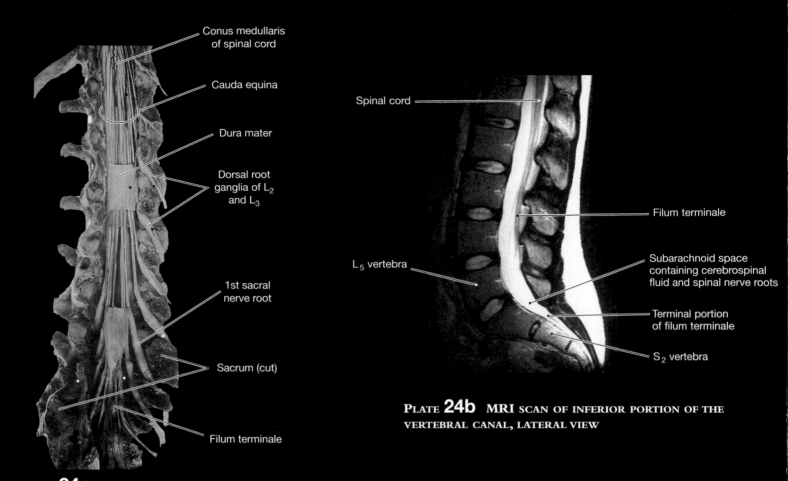

Conus medullaris
of spinal cord

Cauda equina

Dura mater

Dorsal root
ganglia of L_2
and L_3

Spinal cord

Filum terminale

L_5 vertebra

Subarachnoid space
containing cerebrospinal
fluid and spinal nerve roots

1st sacral
nerve root

Terminal portion
of filum terminale

S_2 vertebra

Sacrum (cut)

PLATE 24b MRI SCAN OF INFERIOR PORTION OF THE
VERTEBRAL CANAL, LATERAL VIEW

Filum terminale

PLATE 24a THE INFERIOR PORTION OF THE
VERTEBRAL COLUMN, POSTERIOR VIEW

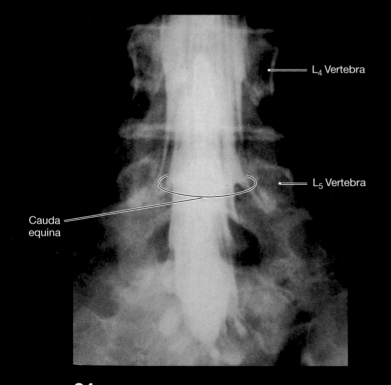

L_4 Vertebra

L_5 Vertebra

Cauda
equina

PLATE 24c X-RAY OF THE CAUDA EQUINA WITH A
CONTRAST MEDIUM IN THE SUBARACHNOID SPACE

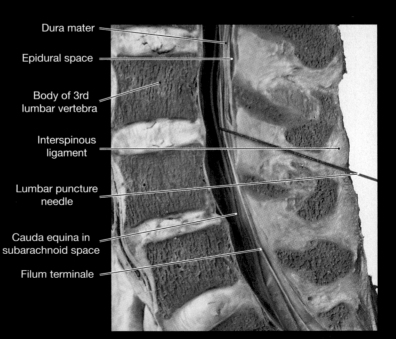

Dura mater

Epidural space

Body of 3rd
lumbar vertebra

Interspinous
ligament

Lumbar puncture
needle

Cauda equina in
subarachnoid space

Filum terminale

PLATE 24d LUMBAR PUNCTURE POSITIONING, SEEN IN A
SAGITTAL SECTION

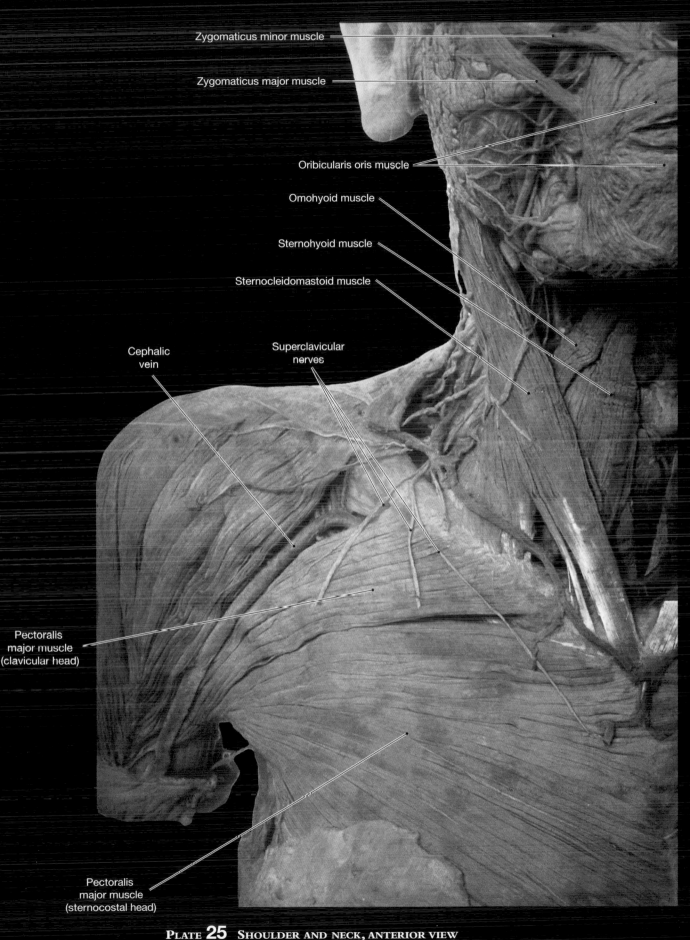

Zygomaticus minor muscle

Zygomaticus major muscle

Oribicularis oris muscle

Omohyoid muscle

Sternohyoid muscle

Sternocleidomastoid muscle

Cephalic vein

Superclavicular nerves

Pectoralis major muscle (clavicular head)

Pectoralis major muscle (sternocostal head)

PLATE 25 SHOULDER AND NECK, ANTERIOR VIEW

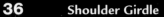

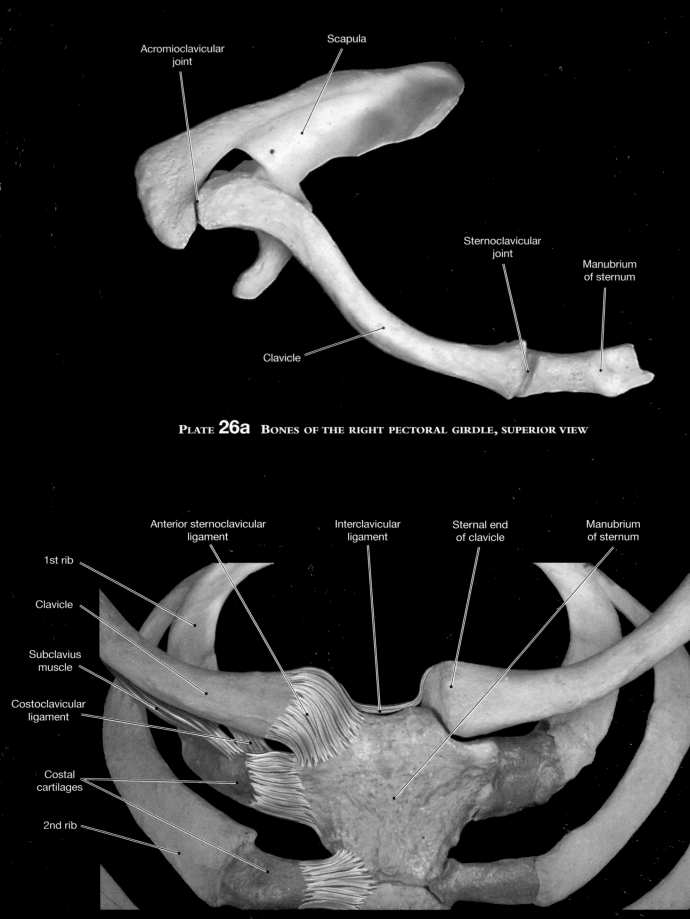

Acromioclavicular joint

Scapula

Sternoclavicular joint

Manubrium of sternum

Clavicle

PLATE 26a BONES OF THE RIGHT PECTORAL GIRDLE, SUPERIOR VIEW

Anterior sternoclavicular ligament

Interclavicular ligament

Sternal end of clavicle

Manubrium of sternum

1st rib

Clavicle

Subclavius muscle

Costoclavicular ligament

Costal cartilages

2nd rib

PLATE 26b STERNOCLAVICULAR JOINT

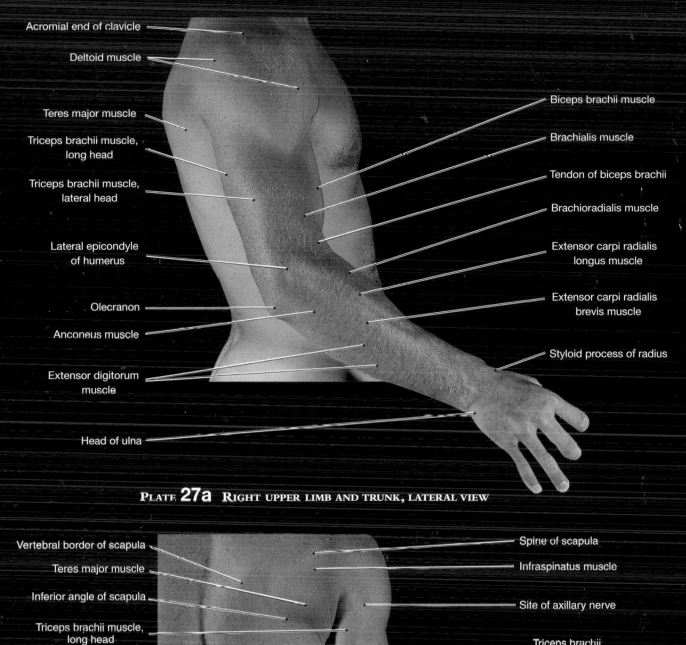

Acromial end of clavicle

Deltoid muscle

Teres major muscle

Triceps brachii muscle, long head

Triceps brachii muscle, lateral head

Lateral epicondyle of humerus

Olecranon

Anconeus muscle

Extensor digitorum muscle

Head of ulna

Biceps brachii muscle

Brachialis muscle

Tendon of biceps brachii

Brachioradialis muscle

Extensor carpi radialis longus muscle

Extensor carpi radialis brevis muscle

Styloid process of radius

PLATE 27a RIGHT UPPER LIMB AND TRUNK, LATERAL VIEW

Vertebral border of scapula

Teres major muscle

Inferior angle of scapula

Triceps brachii muscle, long head

Triceps brachii muscle, medial head

Tendon of insertion of triceps brachii

Medial epicondyle of humerus

Site of palpation for ulnar nerve

Olecranon

Anconeus muscle

Extensor carpi ulnaris muscle

Flexor carpi ulnaris muscle

Spine of scapula

Infraspinatus muscle

Site of axillary nerve

Triceps brachii muscle, lateral head

Brachioradialis muscle

Extensor carpi radialis longus muscle

Extensor carpi radialis brevis muscle

Extensor digitorum muscle

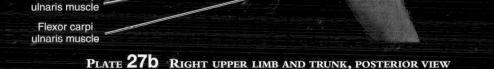

PLATE 27b RIGHT UPPER LIMB AND TRUNK, POSTERIOR VIEW

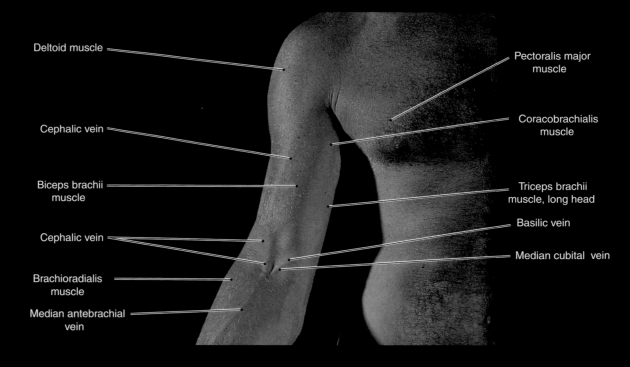

Deltoid muscle

Cephalic vein

Biceps brachii muscle

Cephalic vein

Brachioradialis muscle

Median antebrachial vein

Pectoralis major muscle

Coracobrachialis muscle

Triceps brachii muscle, long head

Basilic vein

Median cubital vein

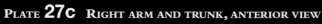

PLATE **27c** RIGHT ARM AND TRUNK, ANTERIOR VIEW

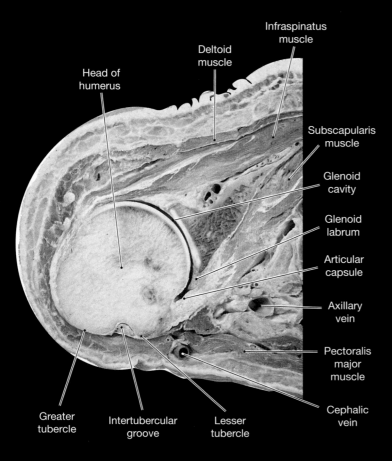

Infraspinatus muscle

Deltoid muscle

Head of humerus

Subscapularis muscle

Glenoid cavity

Glenoid labrum

Articular capsule

Axillary vein

Pectoralis major muscle

Cephalic vein

Greater tubercle

Intertubercular groove

Lesser tubercle

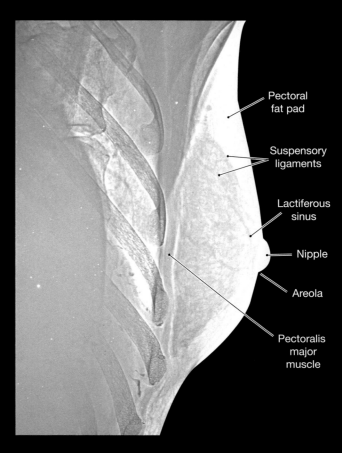

Pectoral fat pad

Suspensory ligaments

Lactiferous sinus

Nipple

Areola

Pectoralis major muscle

PLATE **27d** HORIZONTAL SECTION THROUGH THE RIGHT SHOULDER

PLATE **28** XEROMAMMOGRAM

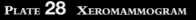

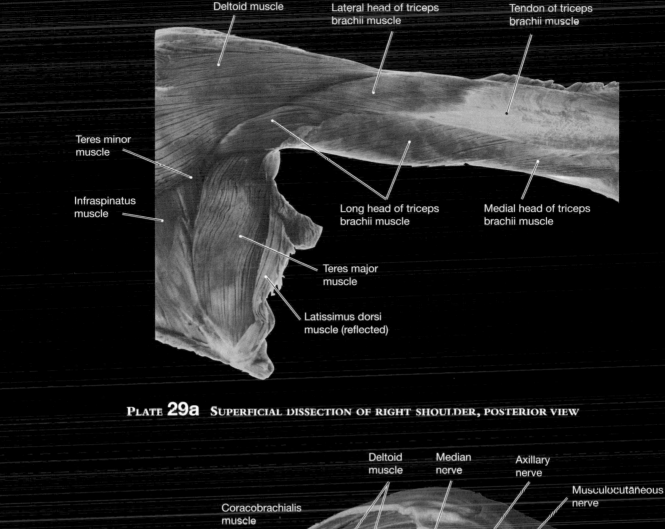

Deltoid muscle

Lateral head of triceps brachii muscle

Tendon of triceps brachii muscle

Teres minor muscle

Infraspinatus muscle

Long head of triceps brachii muscle

Medial head of triceps brachii muscle

Teres major muscle

Latissimus dorsi muscle (reflected)

PLATE 29a SUPERFICIAL DISSECTION OF RIGHT SHOULDER, POSTERIOR VIEW

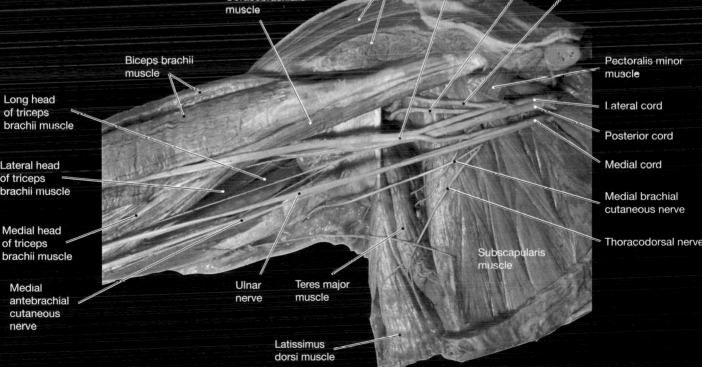

Deltoid muscle

Median nerve

Axillary nerve

Musculocutaneous nerve

Coracobrachialis muscle

Biceps brachii muscle

Pectoralis minor muscle

Long head of triceps brachii muscle

Lateral cord

Posterior cord

Lateral head of triceps brachii muscle

Medial cord

Medial brachial cutaneous nerve

Medial head of triceps brachii muscle

Thoracodorsal nerve

Subscapularis muscle

Medial antebrachial cutaneous nerve

Ulnar nerve

Teres major muscle

Latissimus dorsi muscle

PLATE 29b DEEP DISSECTION OF THE RIGHT BRACHIAL PLEXUS

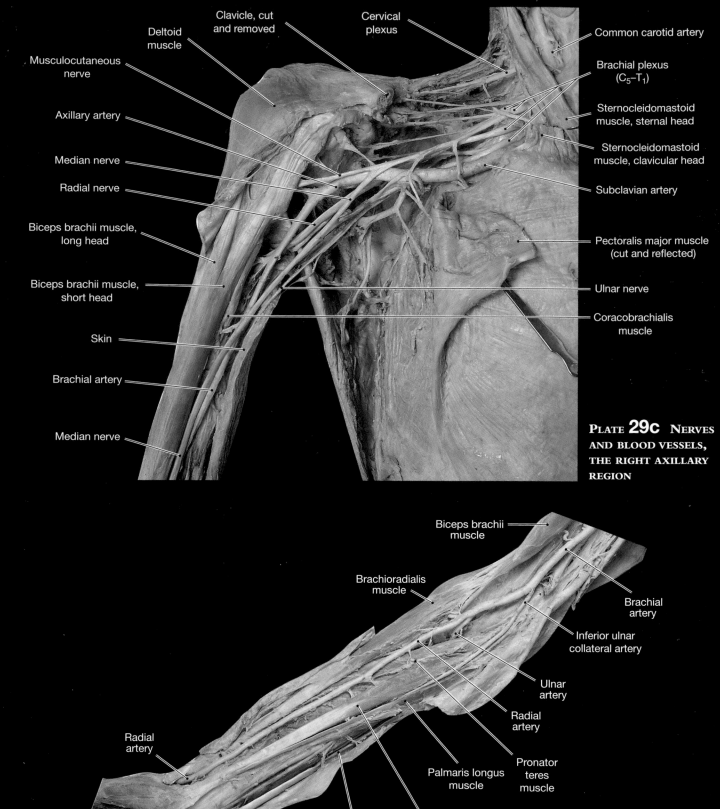

Deltoid muscle

Clavicle, cut and removed

Cervical plexus

Common carotid artery

Musculocutaneous nerve

Brachial plexus (C₅–T₁)

Sternocleidomastoid muscle, sternal head

Axillary artery

Sternocleidomastoid muscle, clavicular head

Median nerve

Radial nerve

Subclavian artery

Biceps brachii muscle, long head

Pectoralis major muscle (cut and reflected)

Biceps brachii muscle, short head

Ulnar nerve

Coracobrachialis muscle

Skin

Brachial artery

Median nerve

PLATE **29c** NERVES AND BLOOD VESSELS, THE RIGHT AXILLARY REGION

Biceps brachii muscle

Brachioradialis muscle

Brachial artery

Inferior ulnar collateral artery

Ulnar artery

Radial artery

Radial artery

Pronator teres muscle

Palmaris longus muscle

Ulnar artery

Flexor carpi ulnaris muscle

Flexor carpi radialis muscle

Superficial palmar arch

PLATE **30** NERVES AND BLOOD VESSELS, THE RIGHT ARM AND FOREARM

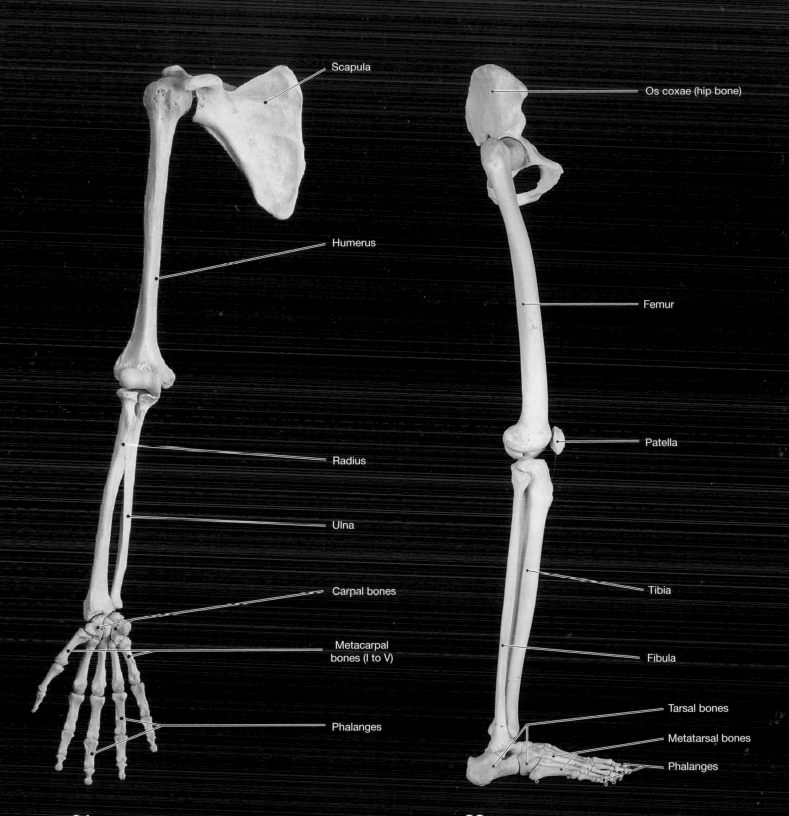

Scapula

Os coxae (hip bone)

Humerus

Femur

Radius

Patella

Ulna

Carpal bones

Tibia

Metacarpal
bones (I to V)

Fibula

Tarsal bones

Metatarsal bones

Phalanges

Phalanges

PLATE **31** BONES OF THE RIGHT UPPER LIMB, ANTERIOR
VIEW

PLATE **32** BONES OF THE RIGHT LOWER LIMB, LATERAL
VIEW

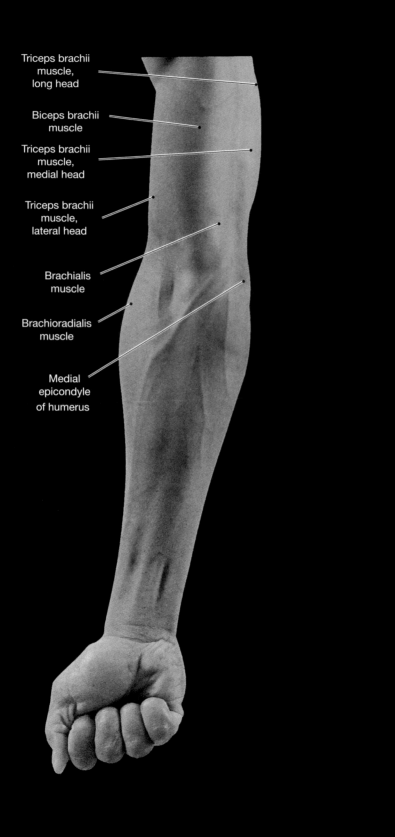

Triceps brachii
muscle,
long head

Biceps brachii
muscle

Triceps brachii
muscle,
medial head

Triceps brachii
muscle,
lateral head

Brachialis
muscle

Brachioradialis
muscle

Medial
epicondyle
of humerus

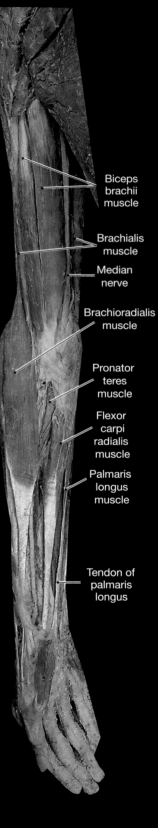

Biceps
brachii
muscle

Brachialis
muscle

Median
nerve

Brachioradialis
muscle

Pronator
teres
muscle

Flexor
carpi
radialis
muscle

Palmaris
longus
muscle

Tendon of
palmaris
longus

PLATE **33a** THE RIGHT UPPER LIMB, ANTERIOR SURFACE,
MUSCLES

PLATE **33b** THE RIGHT UPPER LIMB, ANTERIOR VIEW,
SUPERFICIAL DISSECTION

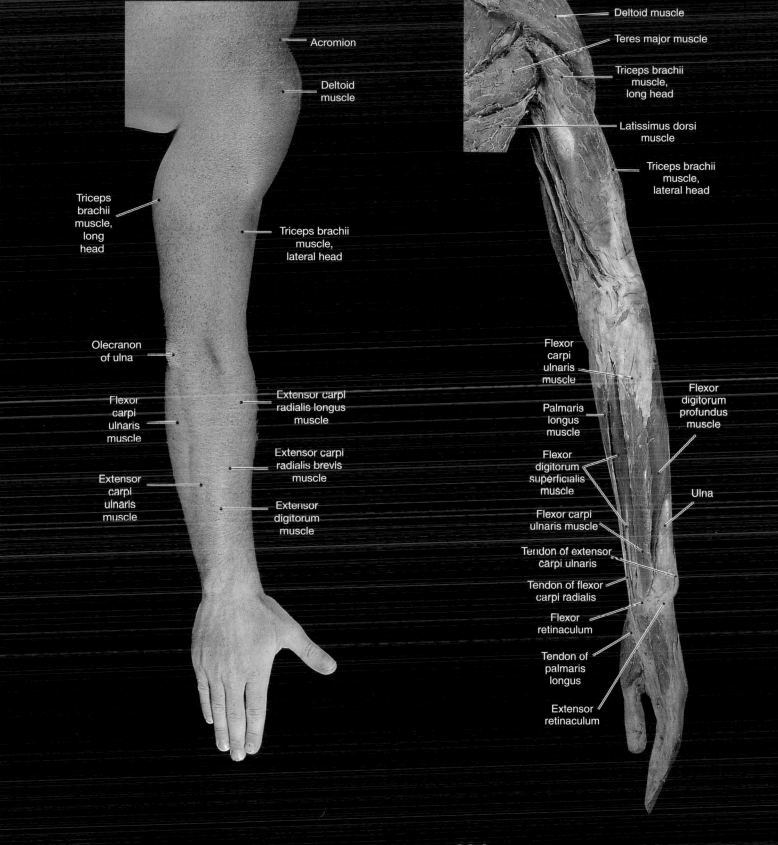

Acromion

Deltoid
muscle

Triceps
brachii
muscle,
long
head

Olecranon
of ulna

Flexor
carpi
ulnaris
muscle

Extensor
carpi
ulnaris
muscle

Triceps brachii
muscle,
lateral head

Extensor carpi
radialis longus
muscle

Extensor carpi
radialis brevis
muscle

Extensor
digitorum
muscle

Deltoid muscle

Teres major muscle

Triceps brachii
muscle,
long head

Latissimus dorsi
muscle

Triceps brachii
muscle,
lateral head

Flexor
carpi
ulnaris
muscle

Palmaris
longus
muscle

Flexor
digitorum
superficialis
muscle

Flexor carpi
ulnaris muscle

Tendon of extensor
carpi ulnaris

Tendon of flexor
carpi radialis

Flexor
retinaculum

Tendon of
palmaris
longus

Extensor
retinaculum

Flexor
digitorum
profundus
muscle

Ulna

PLATE **33c** THE RIGHT UPPER LIMB, POSTERIOR SURFACE,
LANDMARKS

PLATE **33d** THE RIGHT UPPER LIMB, POSTERIOR VIEW,
SUPERFICIAL DISSECTION

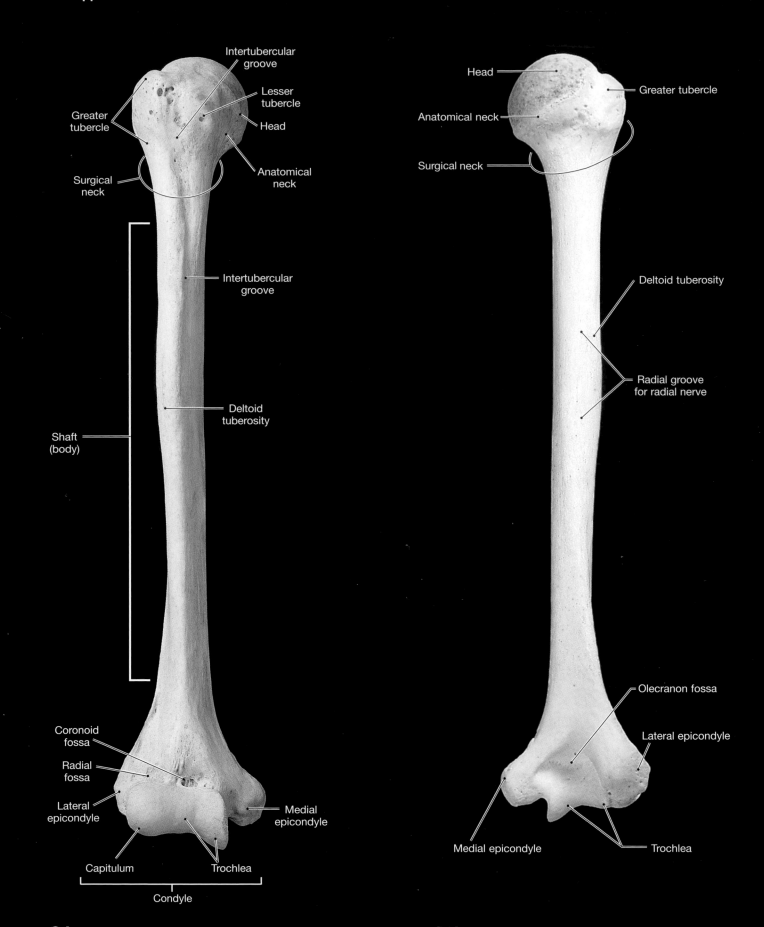

Intertubercular groove

Lesser tubercle

Head

Greater tubercle

Anatomical neck

Surgical neck

Intertubercular groove

Shaft (body)

Deltoid tuberosity

Coronoid fossa

Radial fossa

Lateral epicondyle

Medial epicondyle

Capitulum

Trochlea

Condyle

Head

Greater tubercle

Anatomical neck

Surgical neck

Deltoid tuberosity

Radial groove for radial nerve

Olecranon fossa

Lateral epicondyle

Medial epicondyle

Trochlea

PLATE **34a** RIGHT HUMERUS, ANTERIOR VIEW

PLATE **34b** RIGHT HUMERUS, POSTERIOR VIEW

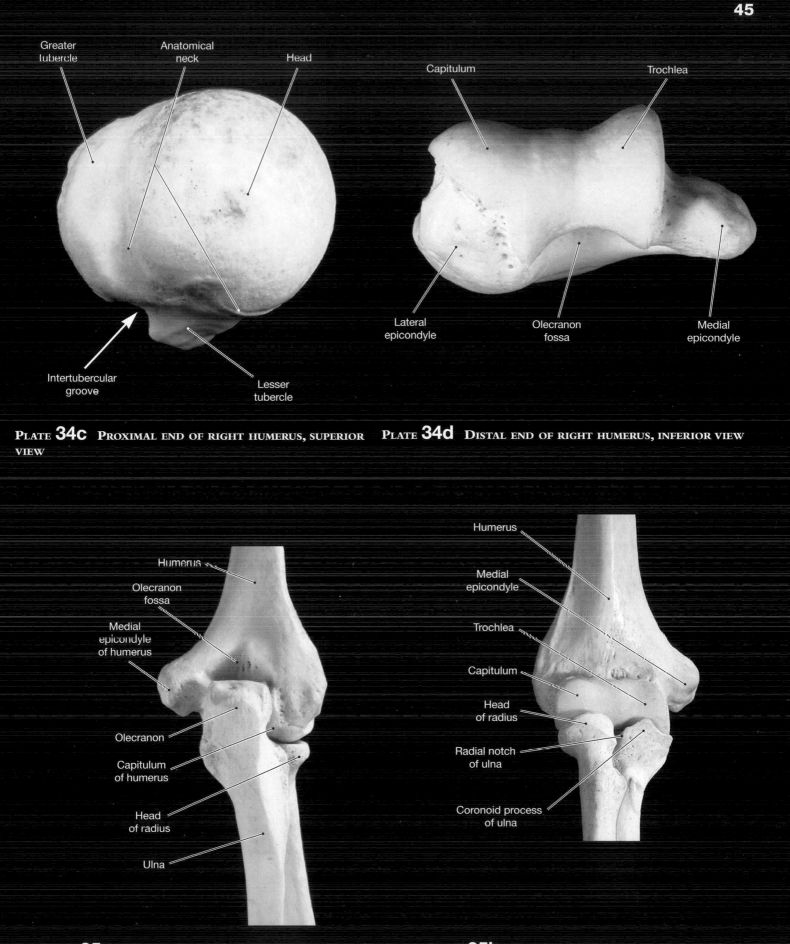

Greater tubercle

Anatomical neck

Head

Capitulum

Trochlea

Intertubercular groove

Lesser tubercle

Lateral epicondyle

Olecranon fossa

Medial epicondyle

PLATE **34c** PROXIMAL END OF RIGHT HUMERUS, SUPERIOR VIEW

PLATE **34d** DISTAL END OF RIGHT HUMERUS, INFERIOR VIEW

Humerus

Olecranon fossa

Medial epicondyle of humerus

Olecranon

Capitulum of humerus

Head of radius

Ulna

Humerus

Medial epicondyle

Trochlea

Capitulum

Head of radius

Radial notch of ulna

Coronoid process of ulna

PLATE **35a** RIGHT ELBOW JOINT, POSTERIOR VIEW

PLATE **35b** RIGHT ELBOW JOINT, ANTERIOR VIEW

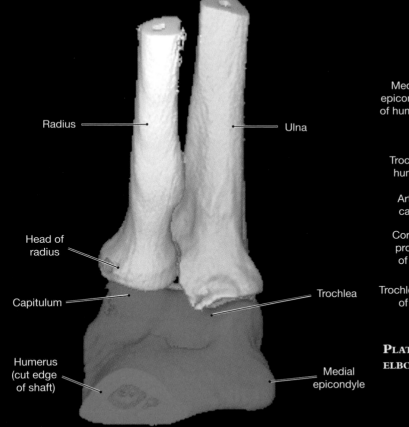

Radius

Ulna

Head of radius

Capitulum

Trochlea

Humerus (cut edge of shaft)

Medial epicondyle

PLATE 35c 3-DIMENSIONAL CT SCAN OF THE RIGHT ELBOW JOINT, SUPERIOR VIEW

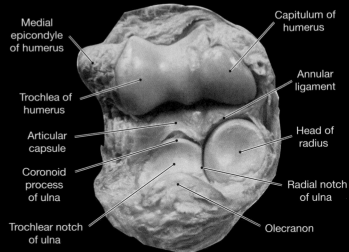

Medial epicondyle of humerus

Capitulum of humerus

Trochlea of humerus

Annular ligament

Articular capsule

Head of radius

Coronoid process of ulna

Radial notch of ulna

Trochlear notch of ulna

Olecranon

PLATE 35e ARTICULAR SURFACES WITHIN THE RIGHT ELBOW JOINT

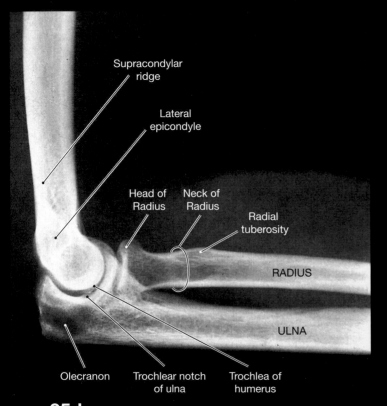

Supracondylar ridge

Lateral epicondyle

Head of Radius

Neck of Radius

Radial tuberosity

RADIUS

ULNA

Olecranon

Trochlear notch of ulna

Trochlea of humerus

PLATE 35d X-RAY OF THE ELBOW JOINT, MEDIAL-LATERAL

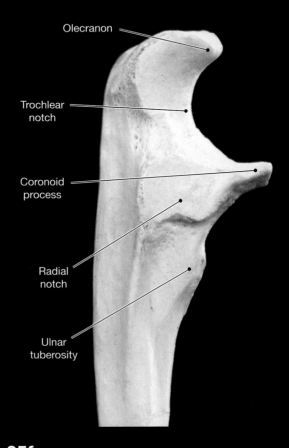

Olecranon

Trochlear notch

Coronoid process

Radial notch

Ulnar tuberosity

PLATE 35f RIGHT ULNA, LATERAL VIEW

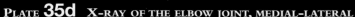

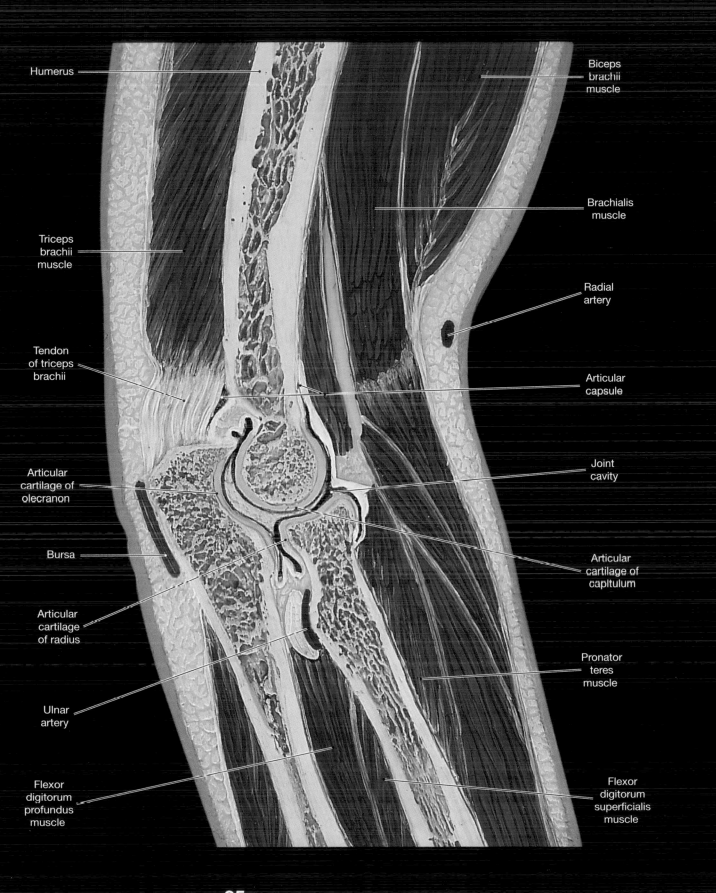

Humerus

Triceps
brachii
muscle

Tendon
of triceps
brachii

Articular
cartilage of
olecranon

Bursa

Articular
cartilage
of radius

Ulnar
artery

Flexor
digitorum
profundus
muscle

Biceps
brachii
muscle

Brachialis
muscle

Radial
artery

Articular
capsule

Joint
cavity

Articular
cartilage of
capltulum

Pronator
teres
muscle

Flexor
digitorum
superficialis
muscle

PLATE **35g** THE ELBOW, OBLIQUE SECTION—MODEL

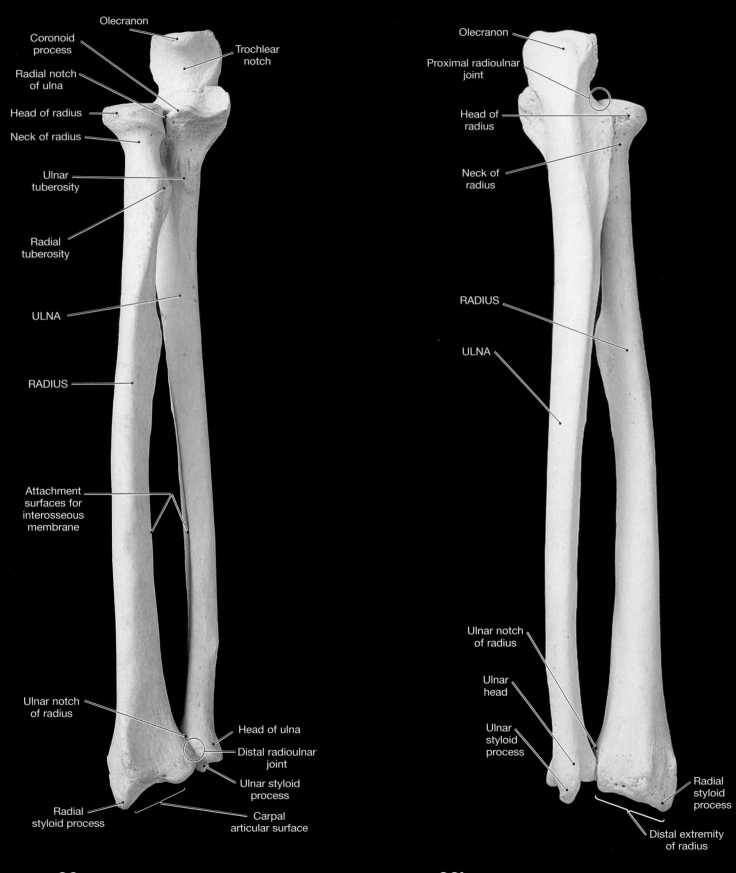

Olecranon

Coronoid
process

Trochlear
notch

Radial notch
of ulna

Head of radius

Neck of radius

Ulnar
tuberosity

Radial
tuberosity

ULNA

RADIUS

Attachment
surfaces for
interosseous
membrane

Ulnar notch
of radius

Head of ulna

Distal radioulnar
joint

Ulnar styloid
process

Radial
styloid process

Carpal
articular surface

Olecranon

Proximal radioulnar
joint

Head of
radius

Neck of
radius

RADIUS

ULNA

Ulnar notch
of radius

Ulnar
head

Ulnar
styloid
process

Radial
styloid
process

Distal extremity
of radius

PLATE **36a** RIGHT RADIUS AND ULNA, ANTERIOR VIEW

PLATE **36b** RIGHT RADIUS AND ULNA, POSTERIOR VIEW

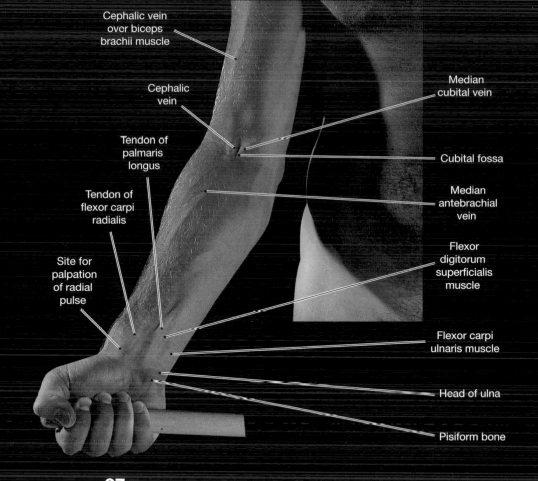

Cephalic vein over biceps brachii muscle

Cephalic vein

Tendon of palmaris longus

Tendon of flexor carpi radialis

Site for palpation of radial pulse

Median cubital vein

Cubital fossa

Median antebrachial vein

Flexor digitorum superficialis muscle

Flexor carpi ulnaris muscle

Head of ulna

Pisiform bone

PLATE **37a** THE RIGHT UPPER LIMB, ANTERIOR SURFACE, LANDMARKS

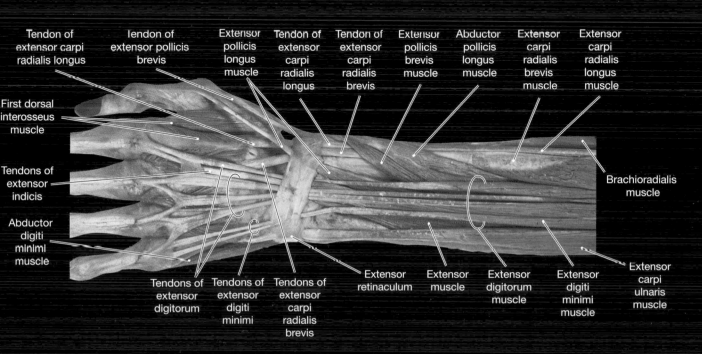

Tendon of extensor carpi radialis longus

Tendon of extensor pollicis brevis

Extensor pollicis longus muscle

Tendon of extensor carpi radialis longus

Tendon of extensor carpi radialis brevis

Extensor pollicis brevis muscle

Abductor pollicis longus muscle

Extensor carpi radialis brevis muscle

Extensor carpi radialis longus muscle

First dorsal interosseus muscle

Tendons of extensor indicis

Abductor digiti minimi muscle

Brachioradialis muscle

Tendons of extensor digitorum

Tendons of extensor digiti minimi

Tendons of extensor carpi radialis brevis

Extensor retinaculum

Extensor muscle

Extensor digitorum muscle

Extensor digiti minimi muscle

Extensor carpi ulnaris muscle

PLATE **37b** SUPERFICIAL DISSECTION OF RIGHT FOREARM AND HAND, POSTERIOR VIEW

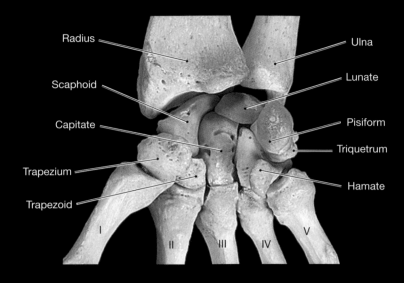

Radius

Ulna

Scaphoid

Lunate

Capitate

Pisiform

Triquetrum

Trapezium

Hamate

Trapezoid

I

II

III

IV

V

PLATE **38a** BONES OF THE RIGHT WRIST, ANTERIOR VIEW

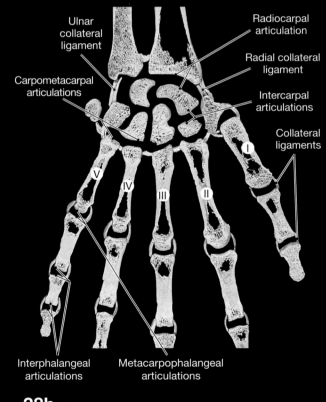

Ulnar
collateral
ligament

Radiocarpal
articulation

Carpometacarpal
articulations

Radial collateral
ligament

Intercarpal
articulations

Collateral
ligaments

I

V

IV

III

II

Interphalangeal
articulations

Metacarpophalangeal
articulations

PLATE **38b** JOINTS OF THE RIGHT WRIST, CORONAL
SECTION

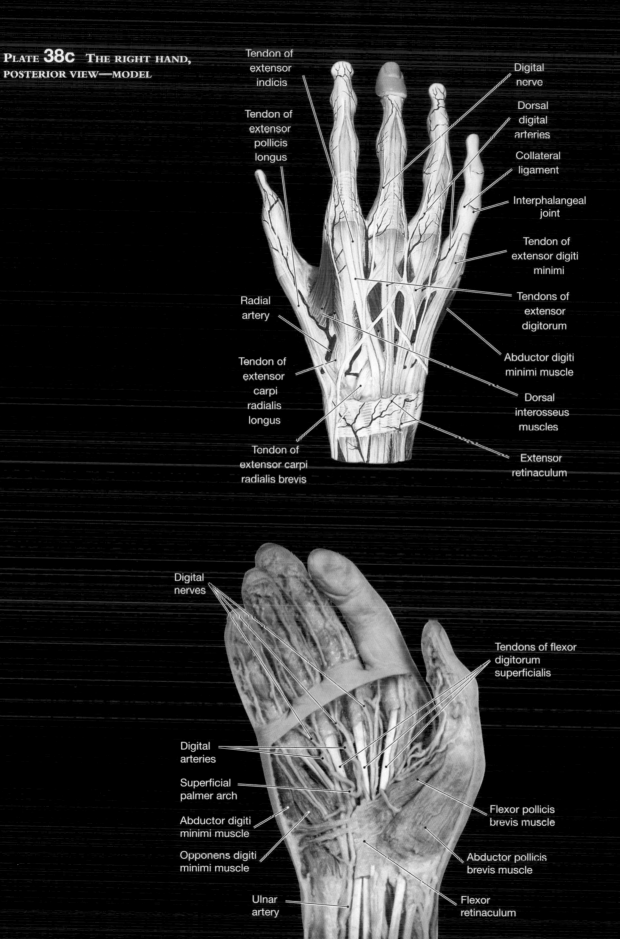

PLATE 38c THE RIGHT HAND, POSTERIOR VIEW—MODEL

Tendon of extensor indicis

Tendon of extensor pollicis longus

Digital nerve

Dorsal digital arteries

Collateral ligament

Interphalangeal joint

Tendon of extensor digiti minimi

Tendons of extensor digitorum

Abductor digiti minimi muscle

Dorsal interosseus muscles

Extensor retinaculum

Radial artery

Tendon of extensor carpi radialis longus

Tendon of extensor carpi radialis brevis

Digital nerves

Tendons of flexor digitorum superficialis

Digital arteries

Superficial palmer arch

Abductor digiti minimi muscle

Opponens digiti minimi muscle

Ulnar artery

Flexor pollicis brevis muscle

Abductor pollicis brevis muscle

Flexor retinaculum

PLATE 38d SUPERFICIAL DISSECTION OF THE RIGHT WRIST AND HAND, ANTERIOR VIEW

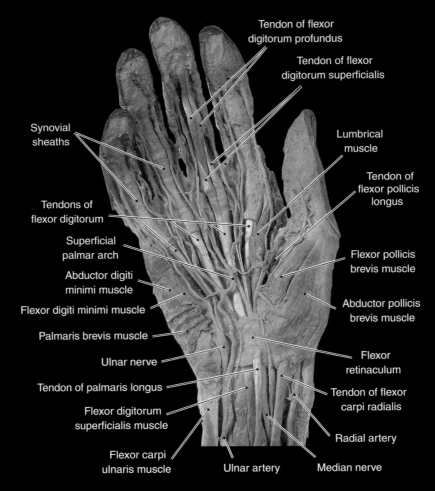

Tendon of flexor
digitorum profundus

Tendon of flexor
digitorum superficialis

Lumbrical
muscle

Tendon of
flexor pollicis
longus

Synovial
sheaths

Tendons of
flexor digitorum

Superficial
palmar arch

Flexor pollicis
brevis muscle

Abductor digiti
minimi muscle

Abductor pollicis
brevis muscle

Flexor digiti minimi muscle

Palmaris brevis muscle

Flexor
retinaculum

Ulnar nerve

Tendon of palmaris longus

Tendon of flexor
carpi radialis

Flexor digitorum
superficialis muscle

Radial artery

Flexor carpi
ulnaris muscle

Ulnar artery

Median nerve

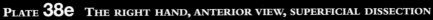

PLATE **38e** THE RIGHT HAND, ANTERIOR VIEW, SUPERFICIAL DISSECTION

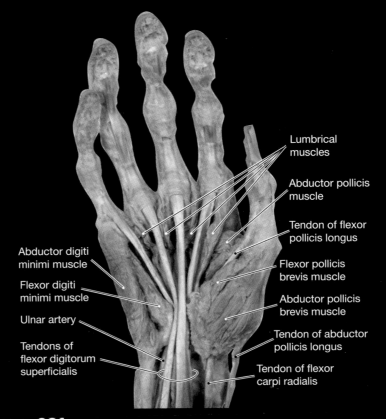

Lumbrical
muscles

Abductor pollicis
muscle

Tendon of flexor
pollicis longus

Flexor pollicis
brevis muscle

Abductor digiti
minimi muscle

Flexor digiti
minimi muscle

Abductor pollicis
brevis muscle

Ulnar artery

Tendon of abductor
pollicis longus

Tendons of
flexor digitorum
superficialis

Tendon of flexor
carpi radialis

PLATE **38f** FLEXOR TENDONS OF RIGHT WRIST AND HAND

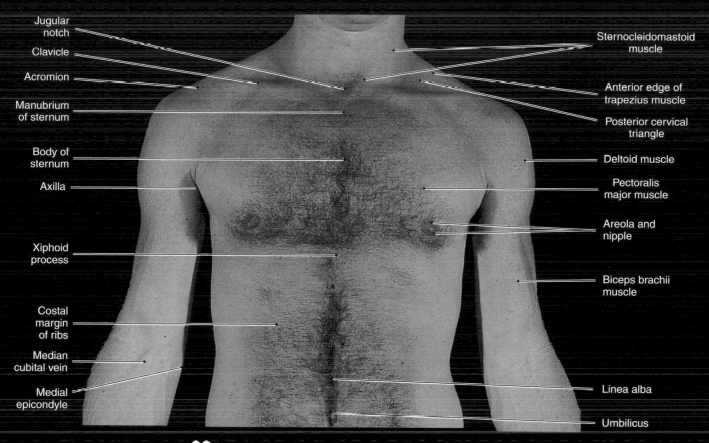

Jugular notch

Clavicle

Acromion

Manubrium of sternum

Body of sternum

Axilla

Xiphoid process

Costal margin of ribs

Median cubital vein

Medial epicondyle

Sternocleidomastoid muscle

Anterior edge of trapezius muscle

Posterior cervical triangle

Deltoid muscle

Pectoralis major muscle

Areola and nipple

Biceps brachii muscle

Linea alba

Umbilicus

PLATE 39a SURFACE ANATOMY OF THE TRUNK, ANTERIOR VIEW

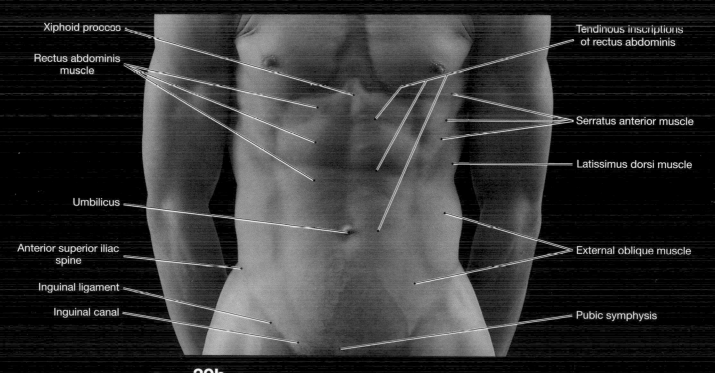

Xiphoid process

Rectus abdominis muscle

Umbilicus

Anterior superior iliac spine

Inguinal ligament

Inguinal canal

Tendinous inscriptions of rectus abdominis

Serratus anterior muscle

Latissimus dorsi muscle

External oblique muscle

Pubic symphysis

PLATE 39b SURFACE ANATOMY OF THE ABDOMEN, ANTERIOR VIEW

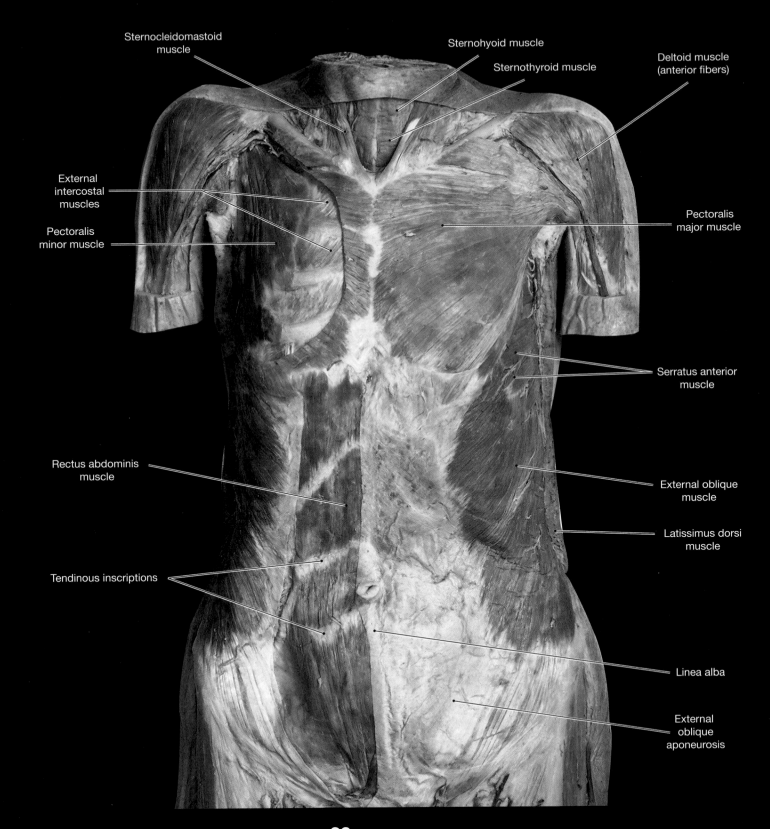

Sternocleidomastoid
muscle

Sternohyoid muscle

Sternothyroid muscle

Deltoid muscle
(anterior fibers)

External
intercostal
muscles

Pectoralis
minor muscle

Pectoralis
major muscle

Serratus anterior
muscle

Rectus abdominis
muscle

External oblique
muscle

Latissimus dorsi
muscle

Tendinous inscriptions

Linea alba

External
oblique
aponeurosis

PLATE **39c**	TRUNK, ANTERIOR VIEW

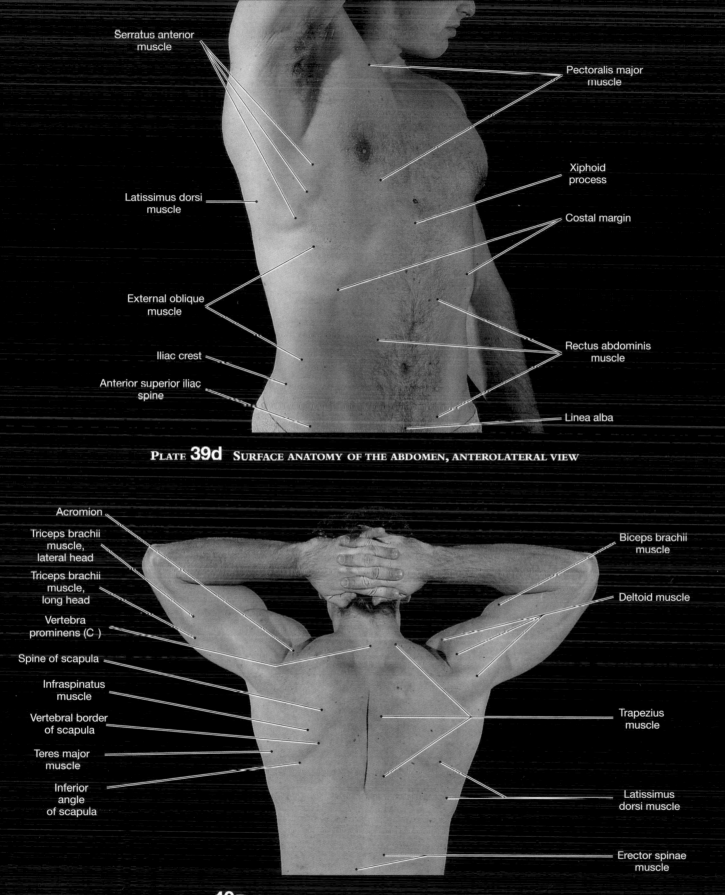

Serratus anterior muscle

Pectoralis major muscle

Xiphoid process

Costal margin

Latissimus dorsi muscle

External oblique muscle

Rectus abdominis muscle

Iliac crest

Anterior superior iliac spine

Linea alba

PLATE **39d** SURFACE ANATOMY OF THE ABDOMEN, ANTEROLATERAL VIEW

Acromion

Biceps brachii muscle

Triceps brachii muscle, lateral head

Triceps brachii muscle, long head

Deltoid muscle

Vertebra prominens (C)

Spine of scapula

Infraspinatus muscle

Trapezius muscle

Vertebral border of scapula

Teres major muscle

Inferior angle of scapula

Latissimus dorsi muscle

Erector spinae muscle

PLATE **40a** SURFACE ANATOMY OF THE TRUNK, POSTERIOR VIEW

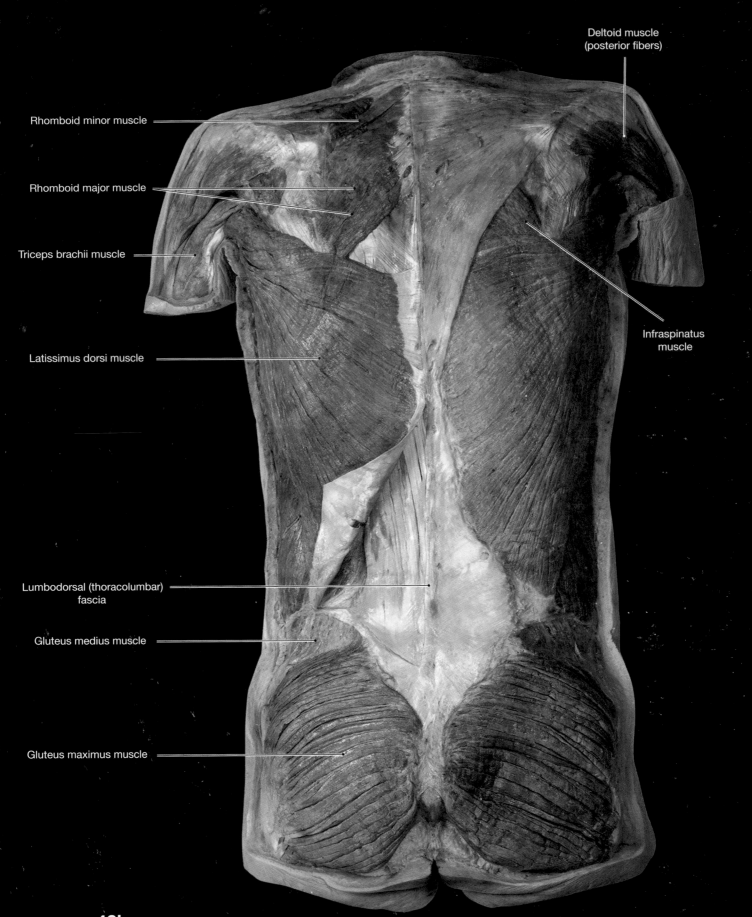

Deltoid muscle
(posterior fibers)

Rhomboid minor muscle

Rhomboid major muscle

Triceps brachii muscle

Latissimus dorsi muscle

Infraspinatus
muscle

Lumbodorsal (thoracolumbar)
fascia

Gluteus medius muscle

Gluteus maximus muscle

PLATE **40b**   TRUNK, POSTERIOR VIEW

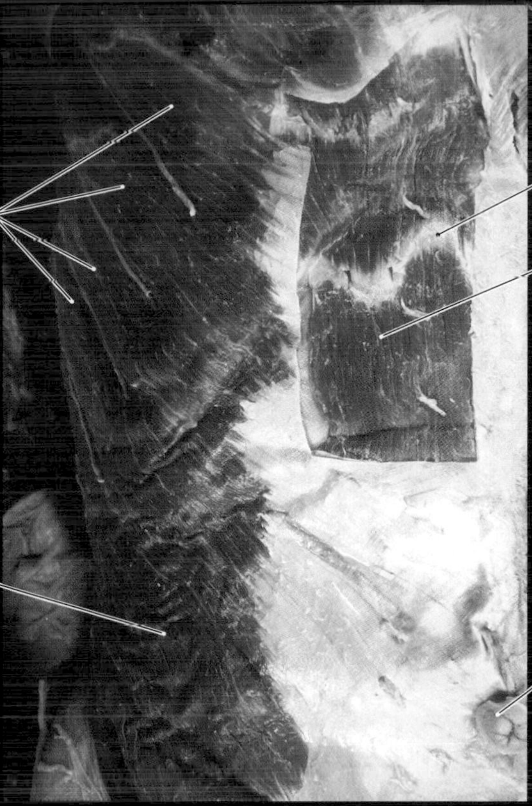

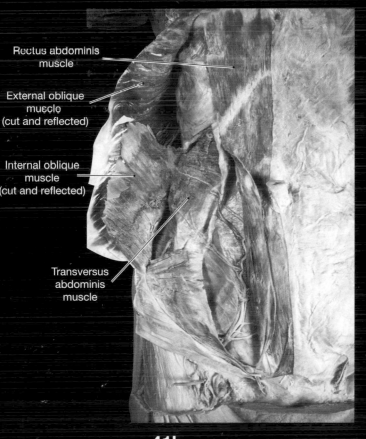

Serratus
anterior
muscle

Tendinous
inscription

Rectus
abdominis
muscle

External
oblique
muscle

Umbilicus

PLATE **41a** ABDOMINAL WALL, ANTERIOR VIEW

Rectus abdominis
muscle

External oblique
muscle
(cut and reflected)

Internal oblique
muscle
(cut and reflected)

Transversus
abdominis
muscle

PLATE **41b** ABDOMINAL MUSCLES

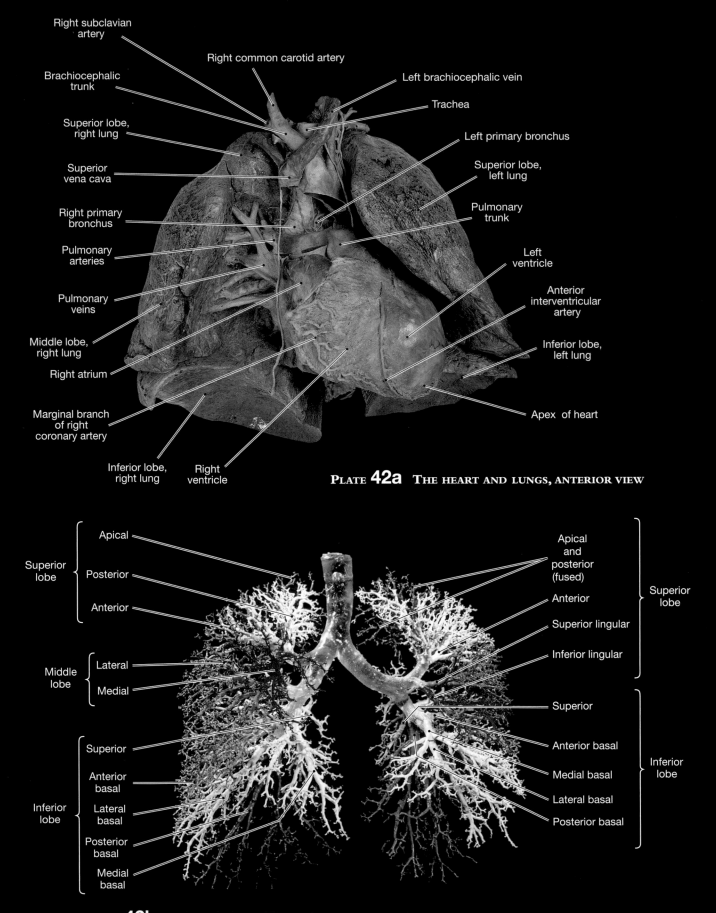

Right subclavian artery

Right common carotid artery

Left brachiocephalic vein

Brachiocephalic trunk

Trachea

Superior lobe, right lung

Left primary bronchus

Superior vena cava

Superior lobe, left lung

Right primary bronchus

Pulmonary trunk

Pulmonary arteries

Left ventricle

Pulmonary veins

Anterior interventricular artery

Middle lobe, right lung

Inferior lobe, left lung

Right atrium

Marginal branch of right coronary artery

Apex of heart

Inferior lobe, right lung

Right ventricle

PLATE 42a   THE HEART AND LUNGS, ANTERIOR VIEW

Apical

Apical and posterior (fused)

Superior lobe

Posterior

Anterior

Anterior

Superior lingular

Inferior lingular

Superior lobe

Middle lobe

Lateral

Medial

Superior

Inferior lobe

Superior

Anterior basal

Anterior basal

Medial basal

Lateral basal

Lateral basal

Inferior lobe

Posterior basal

Posterior basal

Medial basal

PLATE 42b   COLOR-CODED CORROSION CAST OF THE BRONCHIAL TREE, ANTERIOR VIEW

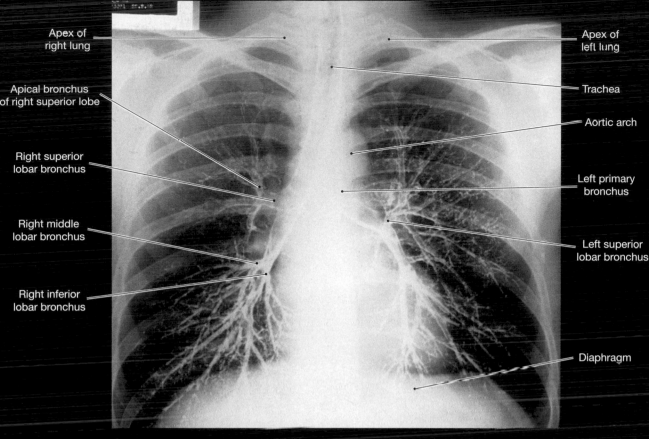

Apex of
right lung

Apex of
left lung

Trachea

Apical bronchus
of right superior lobe

Aortic arch

Right superior
lobar bronchus

Left primary
bronchus

Right middle
lobar bronchus

Left superior
lobar bronchus

Right inferior
lobar bronchus

Diaphragm

PLATE **42c** BRONCHOGRAM

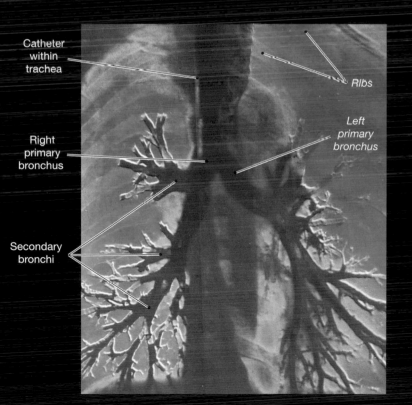

Catheter
within
trachea

Ribs

Right
primary
bronchus

*Left
primary
bronchus*

Secondary
bronchi

PLATE **42d** COLORIZED BRONCHOGRAM

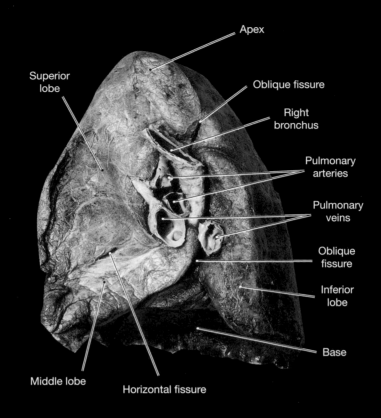

Apex

Superior
lobe

Oblique fissure

Right
bronchus

Pulmonary
arteries

Pulmonary
veins

Oblique
fissure

Inferior
lobe

Base

Middle lobe

Horizontal fissure

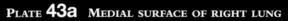

PLATE **43a** MEDIAL SURFACE OF RIGHT LUNG

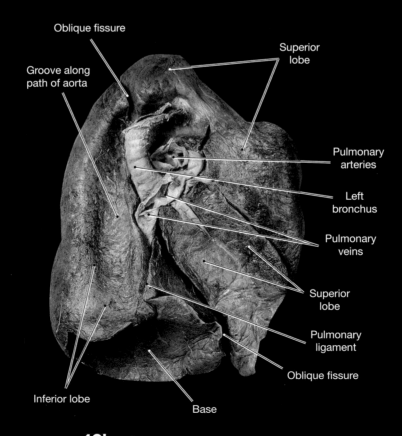

Oblique fissure

Groove along
path of aorta

Superior
lobe

Pulmonary
arteries

Left
bronchus

Pulmonary
veins

Superior
lobe

Pulmonary
ligament

Oblique fissure

Inferior lobe

Base

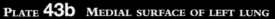

PLATE **43b** MEDIAL SURFACE OF LEFT LUNG

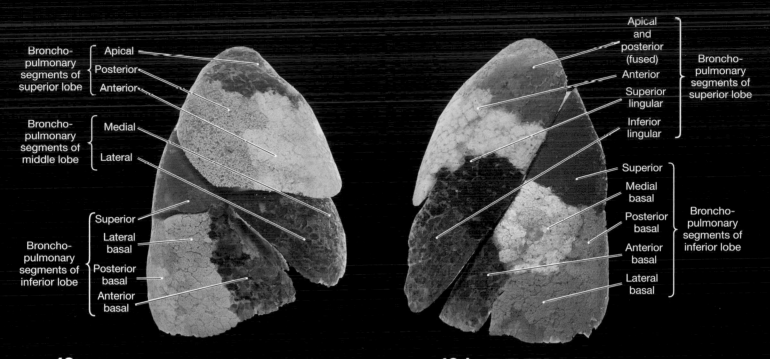

Broncho-pulmonary segments of superior lobe { Apical / Posterior / Anterior

Broncho-pulmonary segments of middle lobe { Medial / Lateral

Broncho-pulmonary segments of inferior lobe { Superior / Lateral basal / Posterior basal / Anterior basal

Apical and posterior (fused) / Anterior / Superior lingular / Inferior lingular } Broncho-pulmonary segments of superior lobe

Superior / Medial basal / Posterior basal / Anterior basal / Lateral basal } Broncho-pulmonary segments of inferior lobe

PLATE 43c BRONCHOPULMONARY SEGMENTS IN THE RIGHT LUNG, LATERAL VIEW

PLATE 43d BRONCHOPULMONARY SEGMENTS IN THE LEFT LUNG, LATERAL VIEW

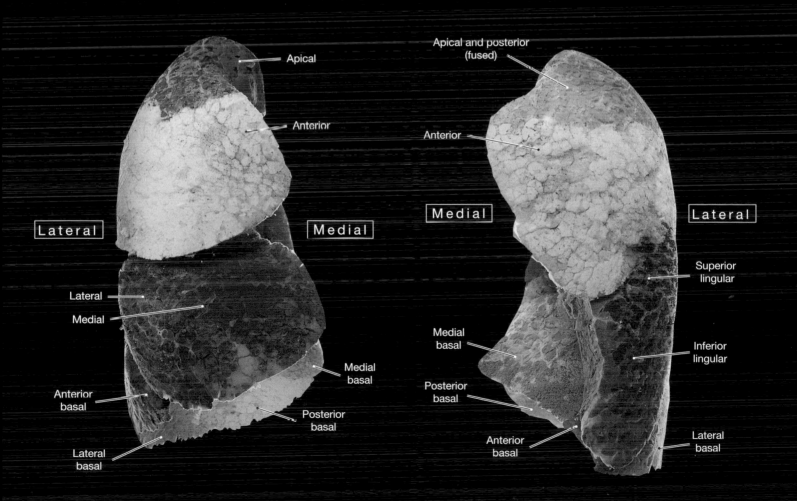

Apical

Anterior

Lateral

Medial

Lateral / Medial

Anterior basal

Medial basal

Posterior basal

Lateral basal

Apical and posterior (fused)

Anterior

Medial / Lateral

Medial basal

Posterior basal

Anterior basal

Superior lingular

Inferior lingular

Lateral basal

PLATE 44a BRONCHOPULMONARY SEGMENTS IN THE RIGHT LUNG, ANTERIOR VIEW

PLATE 44b BRONCHOPULMONARY SEGMENTS IN THE LEFT LUNG, ANTERIOR VIEW

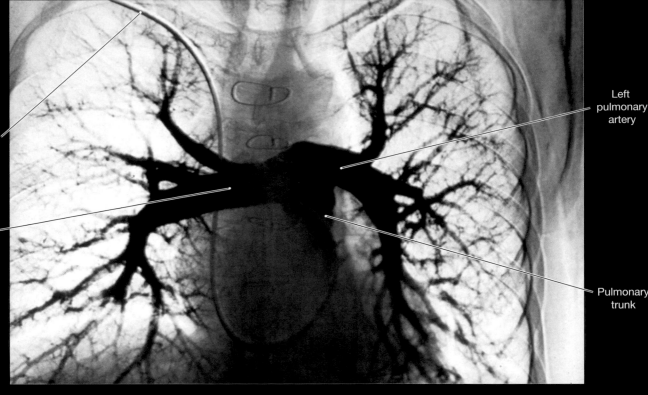

Catheter passing through the right atrium and ventricle to enter the pulmonary trunk

Right pulmonary artery

Left pulmonary artery

Pulmonary trunk

PLATE **44c** PULMONARY ANGIOGRAM

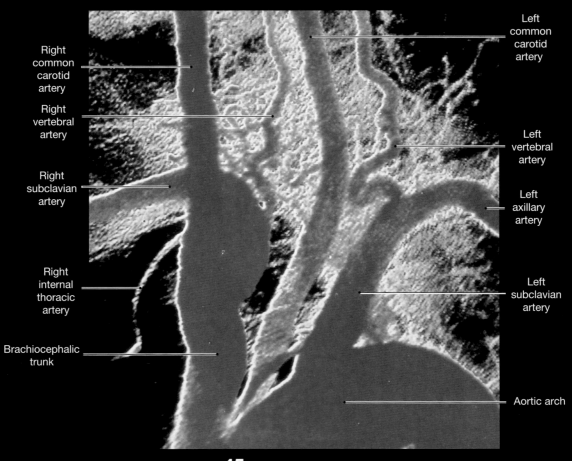

Right common carotid artery

Right vertebral artery

Right subclavian artery

Right internal thoracic artery

Brachiocephalic trunk

Left common carotid artery

Left vertebral artery

Left axillary artery

Left subclavian artery

Aortic arch

PLATE **45a** AORTIC ANGIOGRAM

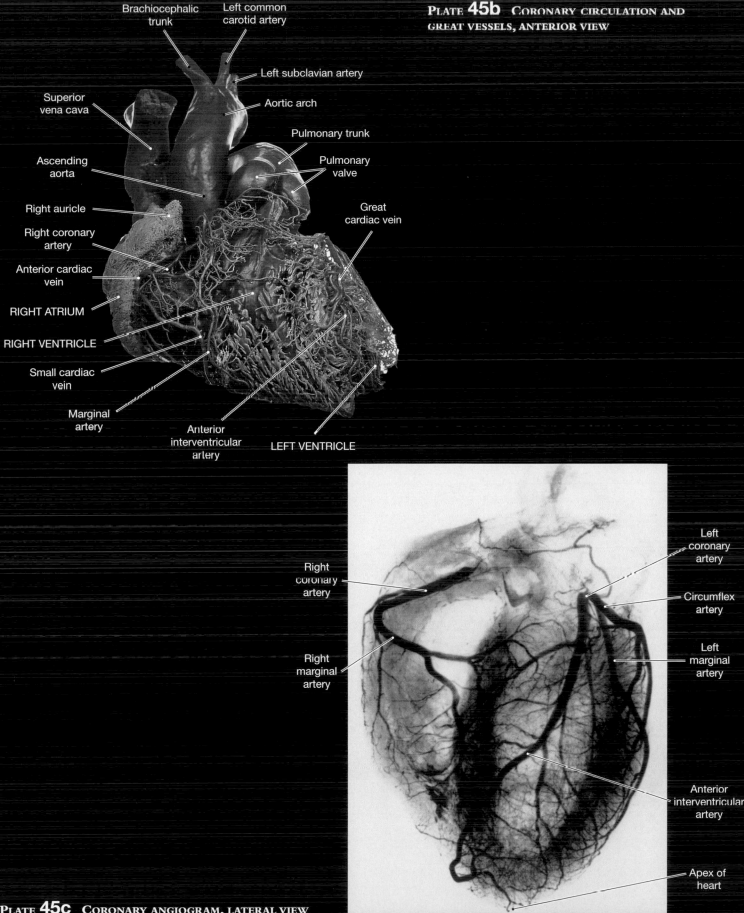

Brachiocephalic trunk

Left common carotid artery

Left subclavian artery

Superior vena cava

Aortic arch

Pulmonary trunk

Pulmonary valve

Ascending aorta

Right auricle

Great cardiac vein

Right coronary artery

Anterior cardiac vein

RIGHT ATRIUM

RIGHT VENTRICLE

Small cardiac vein

Marginal artery

Anterior interventricular artery

LEFT VENTRICLE

Right coronary artery

Left coronary artery

Circumflex artery

Right marginal artery

Left marginal artery

Anterior interventricular artery

Apex of heart

PLATE **45c** CORONARY ANGIOGRAM, LATERAL VIEW

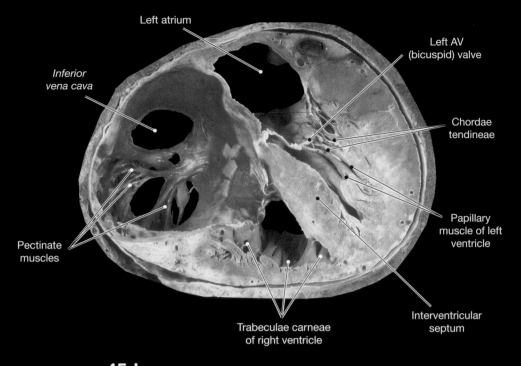

Left atrium

Inferior
vena cava

Left AV
(bicuspid) valve

Chordae
tendineae

Papillary
muscle of left
ventricle

Pectinate
muscles

Trabeculae carneae
of right ventricle

Interventricular
septum

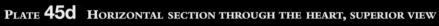

PLATE 45d HORIZONTAL SECTION THROUGH THE HEART, SUPERIOR VIEW

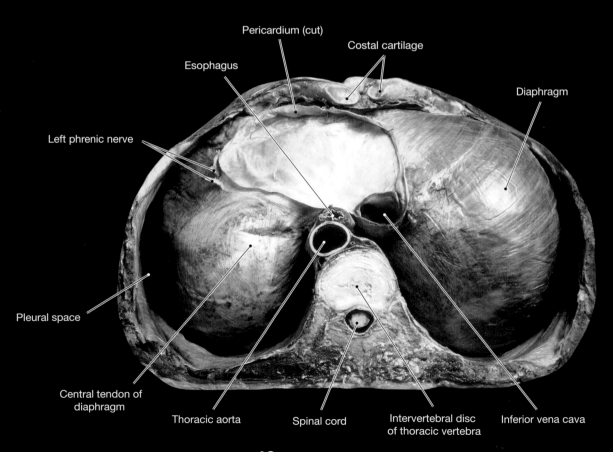

Pericardium (cut)

Costal cartilage

Esophagus

Diaphragm

Left phrenic nerve

Pleural space

Central tendon of
diaphragm

Thoracic aorta

Spinal cord

Intervertebral disc
of thoracic vertebra

Inferior vena cava

PLATE 46 DIAPHRAGM, SUPERIOR VIEW

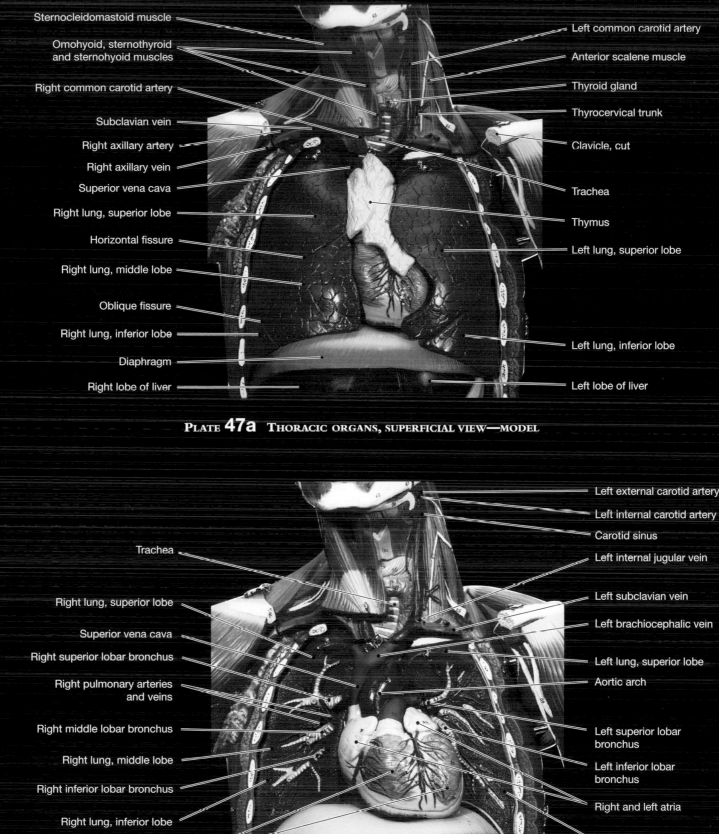

Sternocleidomastoid muscle

Omohyoid, sternothyroid and sternohyoid muscles

Right common carotid artery

Subclavian vein

Right axillary artery

Right axillary vein

Superior vena cava

Right lung, superior lobe

Horizontal fissure

Right lung, middle lobe

Oblique fissure

Right lung, inferior lobe

Diaphragm

Right lobe of liver

Left common carotid artery

Anterior scalene muscle

Thyroid gland

Thyrocervical trunk

Clavicle, cut

Trachea

Thymus

Left lung, superior lobe

Left lung, inferior lobe

Left lobe of liver

PLATE **47a** THORACIC ORGANS, SUPERFICIAL VIEW—MODEL

Trachea

Right lung, superior lobe

Superior vena cava

Right superior lobar bronchus

Right pulmonary arteries and veins

Right middle lobar bronchus

Right lung, middle lobe

Right inferior lobar bronchus

Right lung, inferior lobe

Right and left ventricles

Left external carotid artery

Left internal carotid artery

Carotid sinus

Left internal jugular vein

Left subclavian vein

Left brachiocephalic vein

Left lung, superior lobe

Aortic arch

Left superior lobar bronchus

Left inferior lobar bronchus

Right and left atria

Left lung, inferior lobe

PLATE **47b** THORACIC ORGANS, INTERMEDIATE VIEW—MODEL

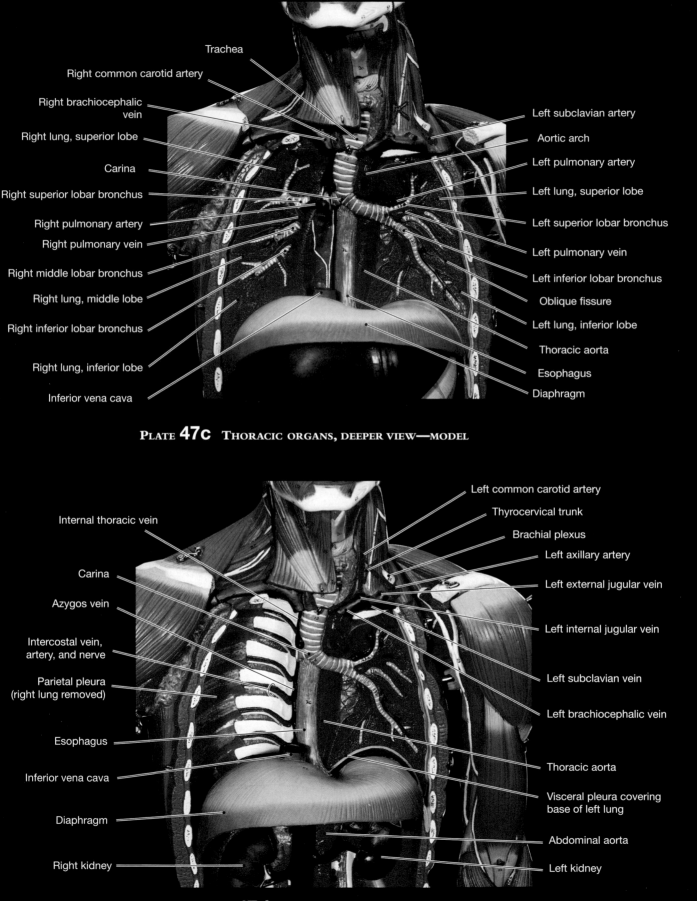

Trachea

Right common carotid artery

Right brachiocephalic vein

Right lung, superior lobe

Carina

Right superior lobar bronchus

Right pulmonary artery

Right pulmonary vein

Right middle lobar bronchus

Right lung, middle lobe

Right inferior lobar bronchus

Right lung, inferior lobe

Inferior vena cava

Left subclavian artery

Aortic arch

Left pulmonary artery

Left lung, superior lobe

Left superior lobar bronchus

Left pulmonary vein

Left inferior lobar bronchus

Oblique fissure

Left lung, inferior lobe

Thoracic aorta

Esophagus

Diaphragm

PLATE **47c** THORACIC ORGANS, DEEPER VIEW—MODEL

Internal thoracic vein

Carina

Azygos vein

Intercostal vein, artery, and nerve

Parietal pleura (right lung removed)

Esophagus

Inferior vena cava

Diaphragm

Right kidney

Left common carotid artery

Thyrocervical trunk

Brachial plexus

Left axillary artery

Left external jugular vein

Left internal jugular vein

Left subclavian vein

Left brachiocephalic vein

Thoracic aorta

Visceral pleura covering base of left lung

Abdominal aorta

Left kidney

PLATE **47d** THE THORACIC CAVITY

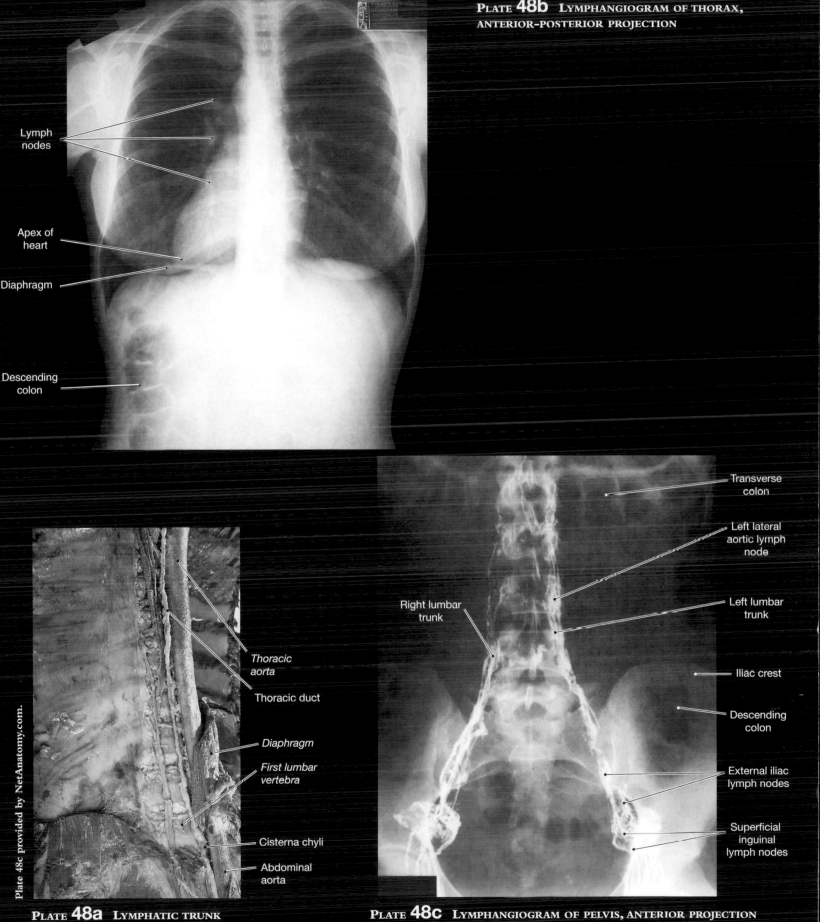

Lymph
nodes

Apex of
heart

Diaphragm

Descending
colon

Transverse
colon

Left lateral
aortic lymph
node

Right lumbar
trunk

Left lumbar
trunk

Iliac crest

Descending
colon

External iliac
lymph nodes

Superficial
inguinal
lymph nodes

Plate 48c provided by NetAnatomy.com.

*Thoracic
aorta*

Thoracic duct

Diaphragm

*First lumbar
vertebra*

Cisterna chyli

Abdominal
aorta

PLATE **48a** LYMPHATIC TRUNK

PLATE **48c** LYMPHANGIOGRAM OF PELVIS, ANTERIOR PROJECTION

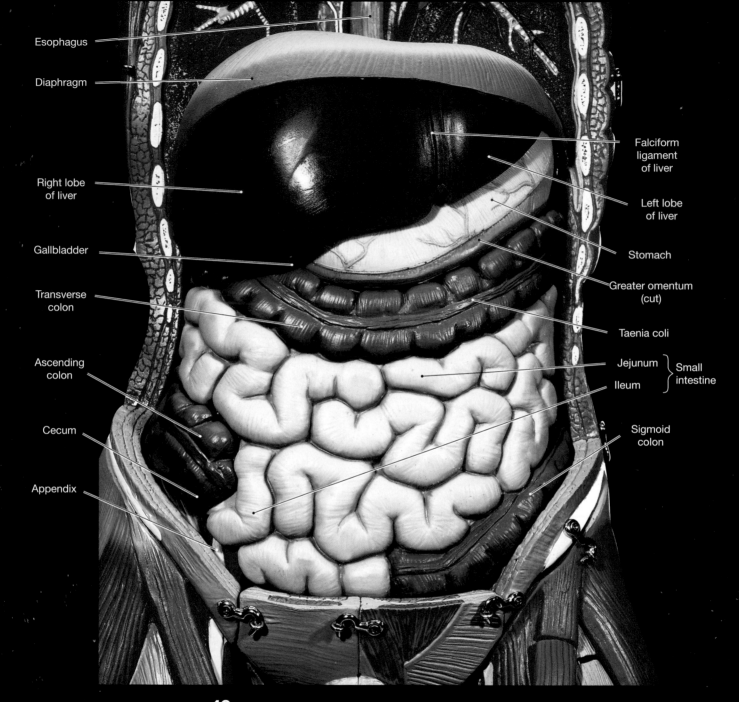

Esophagus

Diaphragm

Right lobe
of liver

Gallbladder

Transverse
colon

Ascending
colon

Cecum

Appendix

Falciform
ligament
of liver

Left lobe
of liver

Stomach

Greater omentum
(cut)

Taenia coli

Jejunum
Ileum } Small
intestine

Sigmoid
colon

PLATE **49a** THE ABDOMINOPELVIC VISCERA, SUPERFICIAL ANTERIOR VIEW

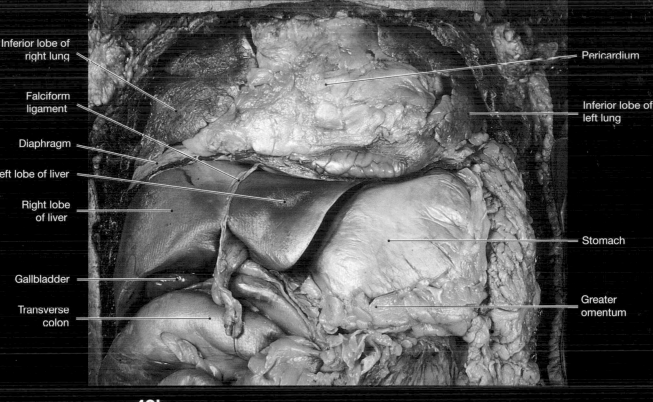

Inferior lobe of right lung

Falciform ligament

Diaphragm

Left lobe of liver

Right lobe of liver

Gallbladder

Transverse colon

Pericardium

Inferior lobe of left lung

Stomach

Greater omentum

PLATE 49b **SUPERIOR PORTION OF ABDOMINOPELVIC CAVITY, ANTERIOR VIEW**

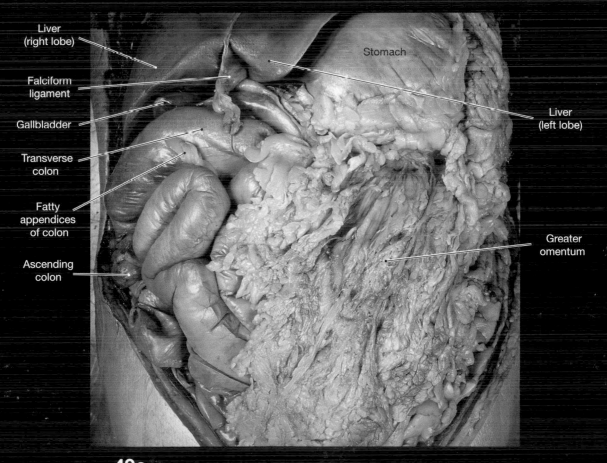

Liver (right lobe)

Falciform ligament

Gallbladder

Transverse colon

Fatty appendices of colon

Ascending colon

Stomach

Liver (left lobe)

Greater omentum

PLATE 49c **INFERIOR PORTION OF ABDOMINOPELVIC CAVITY, ANTERIOR VIEW**

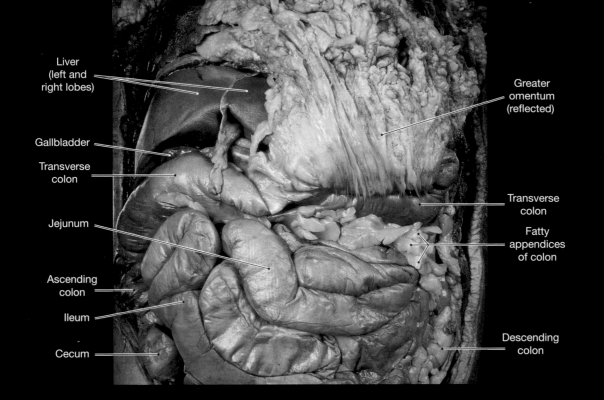

Liver (left and right lobes)

Gallbladder

Transverse colon

Jejunum

Ascending colon

Ileum

Cecum

Greater omentum (reflected)

Transverse colon

Fatty appendices of colon

Descending colon

PLATE **49d** ABDOMINAL DISSECTION, GREATER OMENTUM REFLECTED

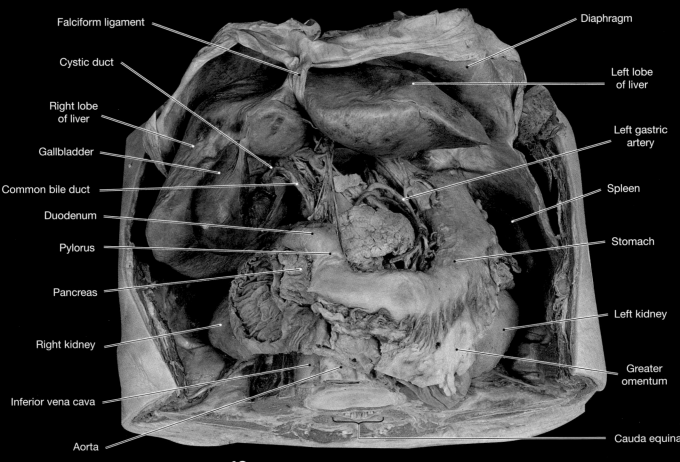

Falciform ligament

Cystic duct

Right lobe of liver

Gallbladder

Common bile duct

Duodenum

Pylorus

Pancreas

Right kidney

Inferior vena cava

Aorta

Diaphragm

Left lobe of liver

Left gastric artery

Spleen

Stomach

Left kidney

Greater omentum

Cauda equina

PLATE **49e** LIVER AND GALLBLADDER IN SITU

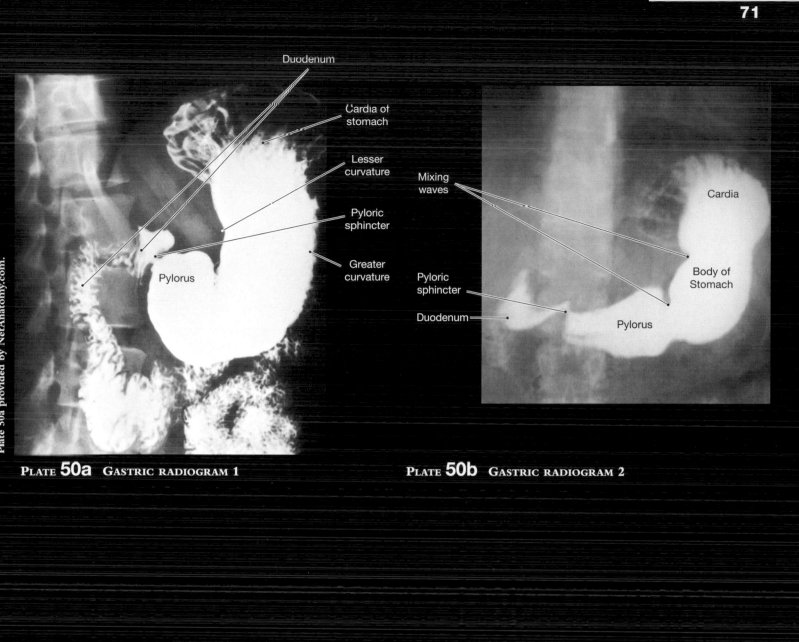

Duodenum

Cardia of
stomach

Lesser
curvature

Pyloric
sphincter

Greater
curvature

Pylorus

PLATE 50a GASTRIC RADIOGRAM 1

Mixing
waves

Cardia

Pyloric
sphincter

Body of
Stomach

Duodenum

Pylorus

PLATE 50b GASTRIC RADIOGRAM 2

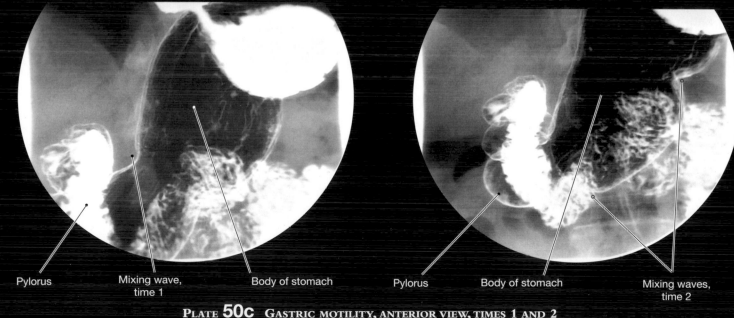

Pylorus

Mixing wave,
time 1

Body of stomach

Pylorus

Body of stomach

Mixing waves,
time 2

PLATE 50c GASTRIC MOTILITY, ANTERIOR VIEW, TIMES 1 AND 2

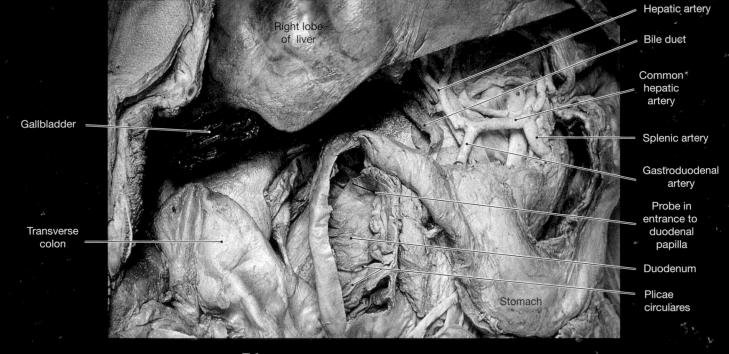

Right lobe
of liver

Hepatic artery

Bile duct

Common
hepatic
artery

Splenic artery

Gastroduodenal
artery

Probe in
entrance to
duodenal
papilla

Duodenum

Plicae
circulares

Gallbladder

Transverse
colon

Stomach

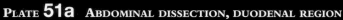

PLATE **51a** ABDOMINAL DISSECTION, DUODENAL REGION

PLATE **51b** GROSS ANATOMY
OF DUODENAL MUCOSA

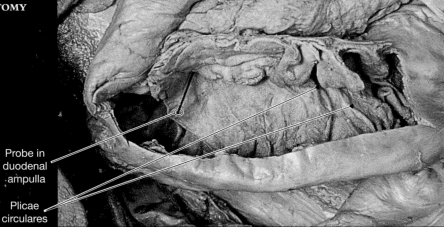

Probe in
duodenal
ampulla

Plicae
circulares

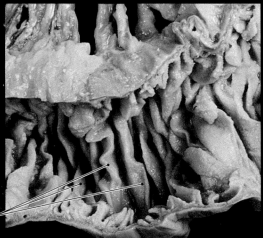

Plicae
circulares

Jejunum

PLATE **51c** GROSS ANATOMY OF THE JEJUNAL MUCOSA

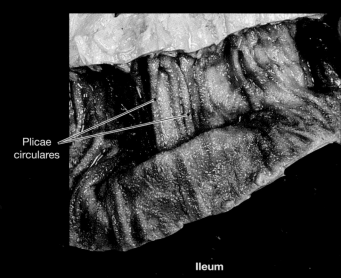

Plicae
circulares

Ileum

PLATE **51d** GROSS ANATOMY OF THE ILEAL MUCOSA

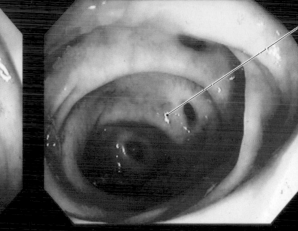

Polyp on wall of colon

Normal section of colon, after removal of a polyp

PLATE 52 NORMAL AND ABNORMAL COLONOSCOPE

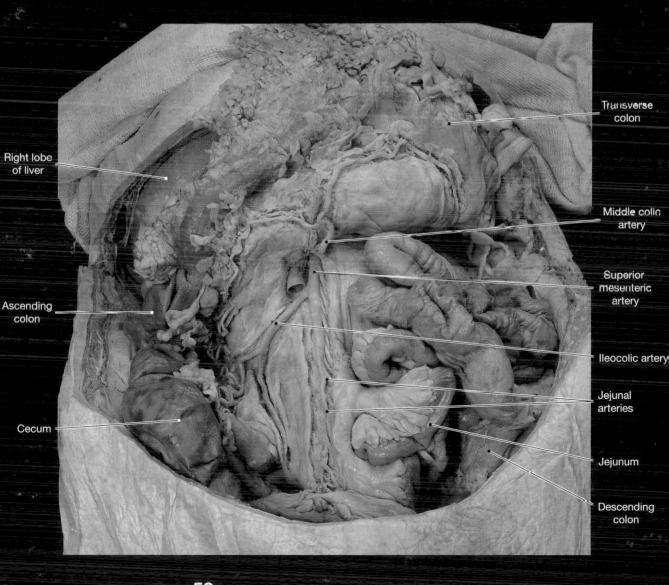

Right lobe of liver

Transverse colon

Middle colic artery

Superior mesenteric artery

Ascending colon

Ileocolic artery

Jejunal arteries

Cecum

Jejunum

Descending colon

PLATE 53a BRANCHES OF THE SUPERIOR MESENTERIC ARTERY

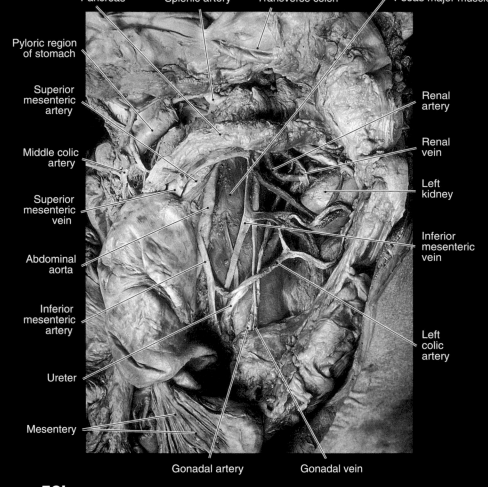

Pancreas   Splenic artery   Transverse colon   Psoas major muscle

Pyloric region
of stomach

Superior
mesenteric
artery

Middle colic
artery

Superior
mesenteric
vein

Abdominal
aorta

Inferior
mesenteric
artery

Ureter

Mesentery

Renal
artery

Renal
vein

Left
kidney

Inferior
mesenteric
vein

Left
colic
artery

Gonadal artery   Gonadal vein

PLATE 53b INFERIOR MESENTERIC VESSELS

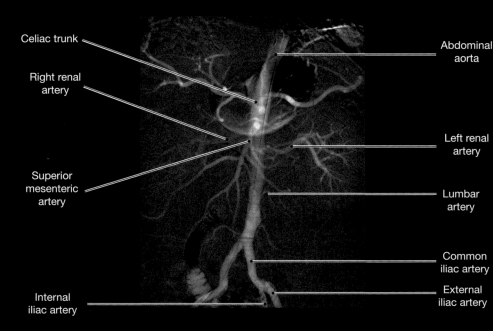

Celiac trunk

Right renal
artery

Superior
mesenteric
artery

Internal
iliac artery

Abdominal
aorta

Left renal
artery

Lumbar
artery

Common
iliac artery

External
iliac artery

PLATE 53c ABDOMINAL ARTERIOGRAM 1

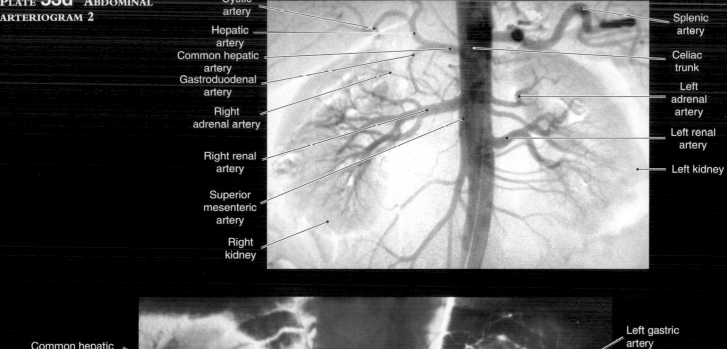

Cystic
artery

Hepatic
artery

Common hepatic
artery

Gastroduodenal
artery

Right
adrenal artery

Right renal
artery

Superior
mesenteric
artery

Right
kidney

Splenic
artery

Celiac
trunk

Left
adrenal
artery

Left renal
artery

Left kidney

Common hepatic
artery

Celiac trunk

Pancreaticoduodenal
artery

Right colic artery

Ileocolic artery

Common iliac
artery

Left gastric
artery

Splenic
artery

Superior
mesenteric
artery

Left
renal
artery

Intestinal
arteries

Terminal
segment of
the aorta

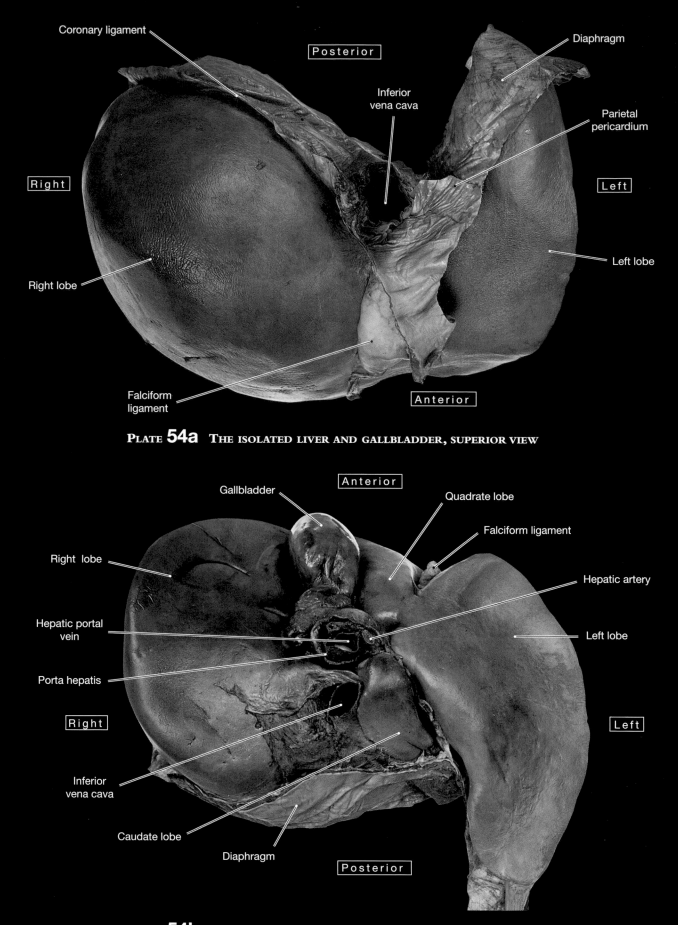

Coronary ligament

Posterior

Inferior vena cava

Diaphragm

Parietal pericardium

Right

Left

Left lobe

Right lobe

Falciform ligament

Anterior

PLATE 54a   THE ISOLATED LIVER AND GALLBLADDER, SUPERIOR VIEW

Anterior

Gallbladder

Quadrate lobe

Falciform ligament

Right lobe

Hepatic artery

Hepatic portal vein

Left lobe

Porta hepatis

Right

Left

Inferior vena cava

Caudate lobe

Diaphragm

Posterior

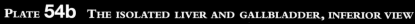

PLATE 54b   THE ISOLATED LIVER AND GALLBLADDER, INFERIOR VIEW

PLATE 54c CORROSION CAST OF LIVER

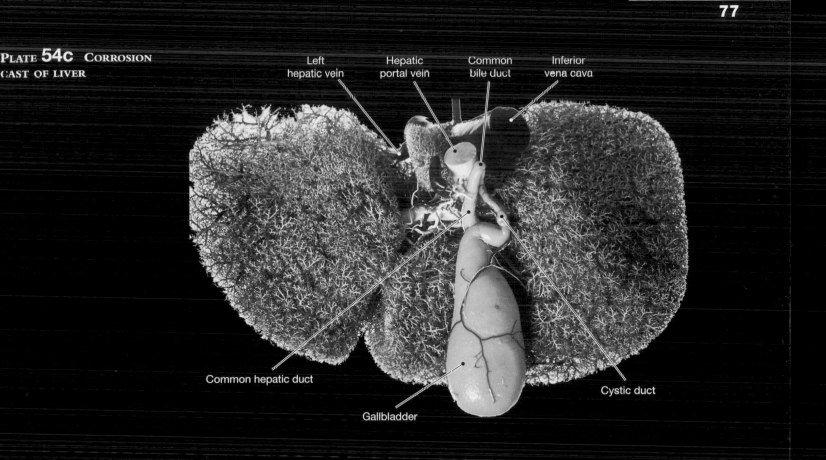

Left hepatic vein

Hepatic portal vein

Common bile duct

Inferior vena cava

Common hepatic duct

Gallbladder

Cystic duct

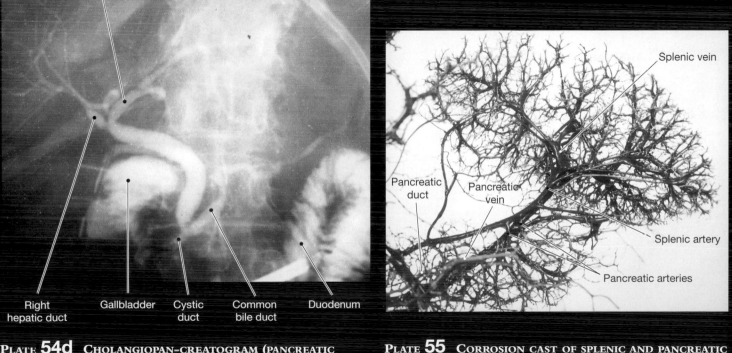

Left hepatic duct

Right hepatic duct

Gallbladder

Cystic duct

Common bile duct

Duodenum

Splenic vein

Pancreatic duct

Pancreatic vein

Splenic artery

Pancreatic arteries

PLATE 54d CHOLANGIOPAN-CREATOGRAM (PANCREATIC

PLATE 55 CORROSION CAST OF SPLENIC AND PANCREATIC

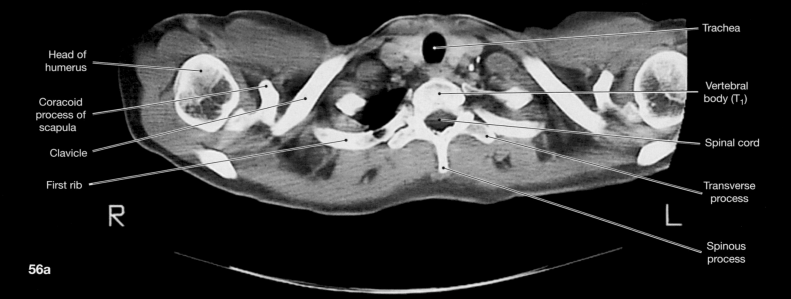

Trachea

Head of humerus

Coracoid process of scapula

Clavicle

First rib

Vertebral body (T₁)

Spinal cord

Transverse process

Spinous process

R

L

56a

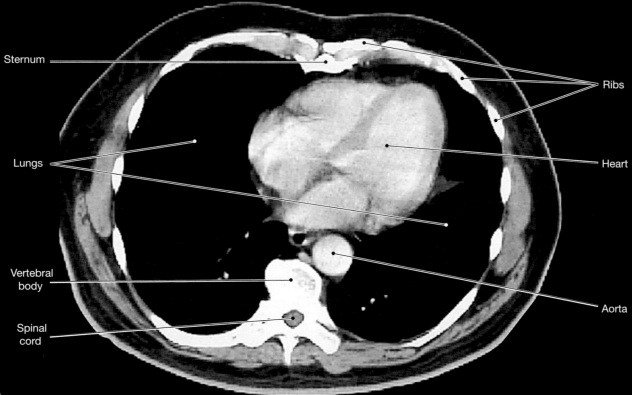

Sternum

Ribs

Lungs

Heart

Vertebral body

Spinal cord

Aorta

56b

PLATES **56a–b** MRI SCANS OF THE TRUNK, HORIZONTAL SECTIONS, SUPERIOR TO INFERIOR SEQUENCE

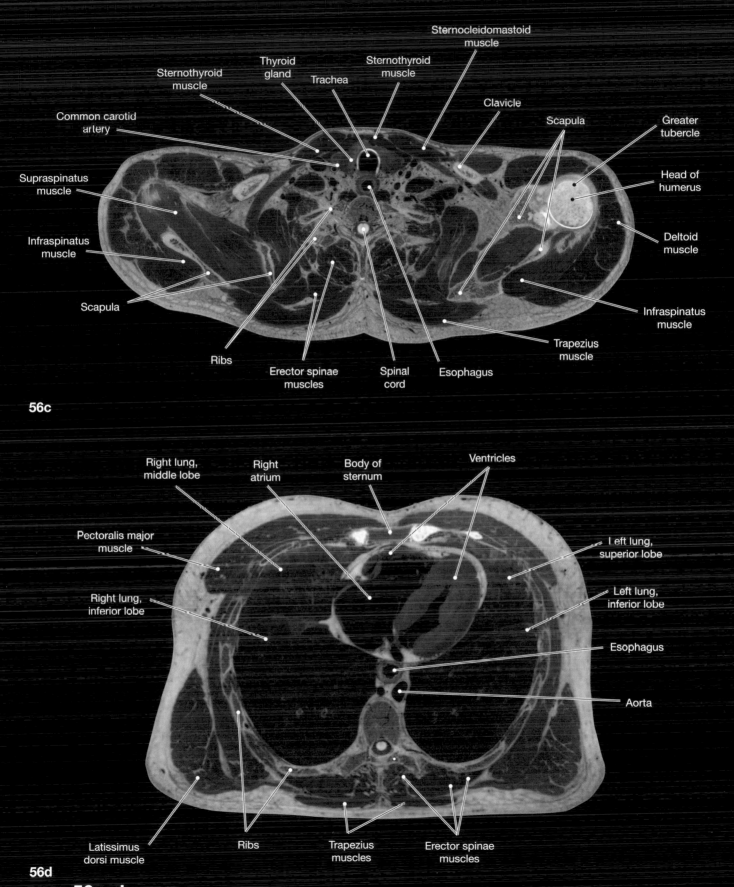

Sternocleidomastoid muscle

Sternothyroid muscle

Thyroid gland

Trachea

Sternothyroid muscle

Clavicle

Scapula

Greater tubercle

Common carotid artery

Head of humerus

Supraspinatus muscle

Deltoid muscle

Infraspinatus muscle

Scapula

Infraspinatus muscle

Ribs

Erector spinae muscles

Spinal cord

Esophagus

Trapezius muscle

56c

Right lung, middle lobe

Right atrium

Body of sternum

Ventricles

Pectoralis major muscle

Left lung, superior lobe

Right lung, inferior lobe

Left lung, inferior lobe

Esophagus

Aorta

Latissimus dorsi muscle

Ribs

Trapezius muscles

Erector spinae muscles

56d

PLATES **56c–d** HORIZONTAL SECTIONS THROUGH THE TRUNK

These sections, derived from the Visible Human dataset, are at the approximate levels of the scans shown in parts a–b.

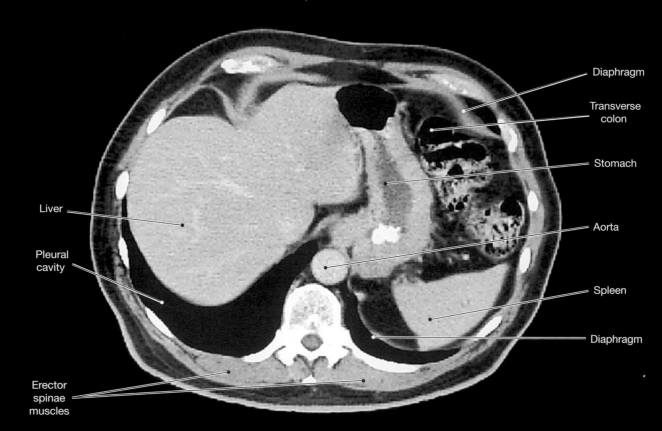

Diaphragm

Transverse
colon

Stomach

Liver

Aorta

Pleural
cavity

Spleen

Diaphragm

Erector
spinae
muscles

56e

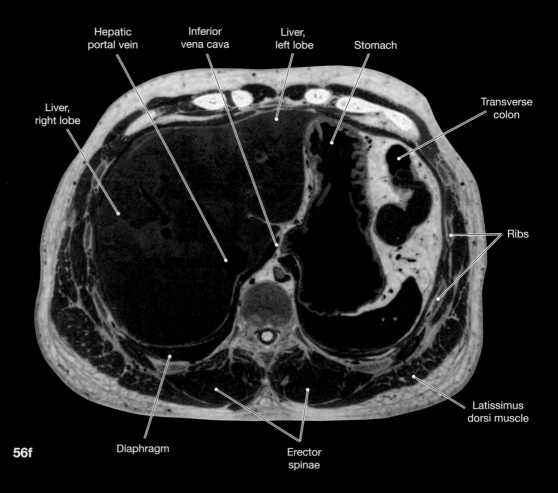

Hepatic
portal vein

Inferior
vena cava

Liver,
left lobe

Stomach

Liver,
right lobe

Transverse
colon

Ribs

Latissimus
dorsi muscle

Diaphragm

Erector
spinae

56f

**PLATES 56e–f HORIZONTAL
SECTIONS THROUGH THE TRUNK**

**Section f, derived from the
Visible Human dataset, is at
the approximate levels of the
scan shown in part e.**

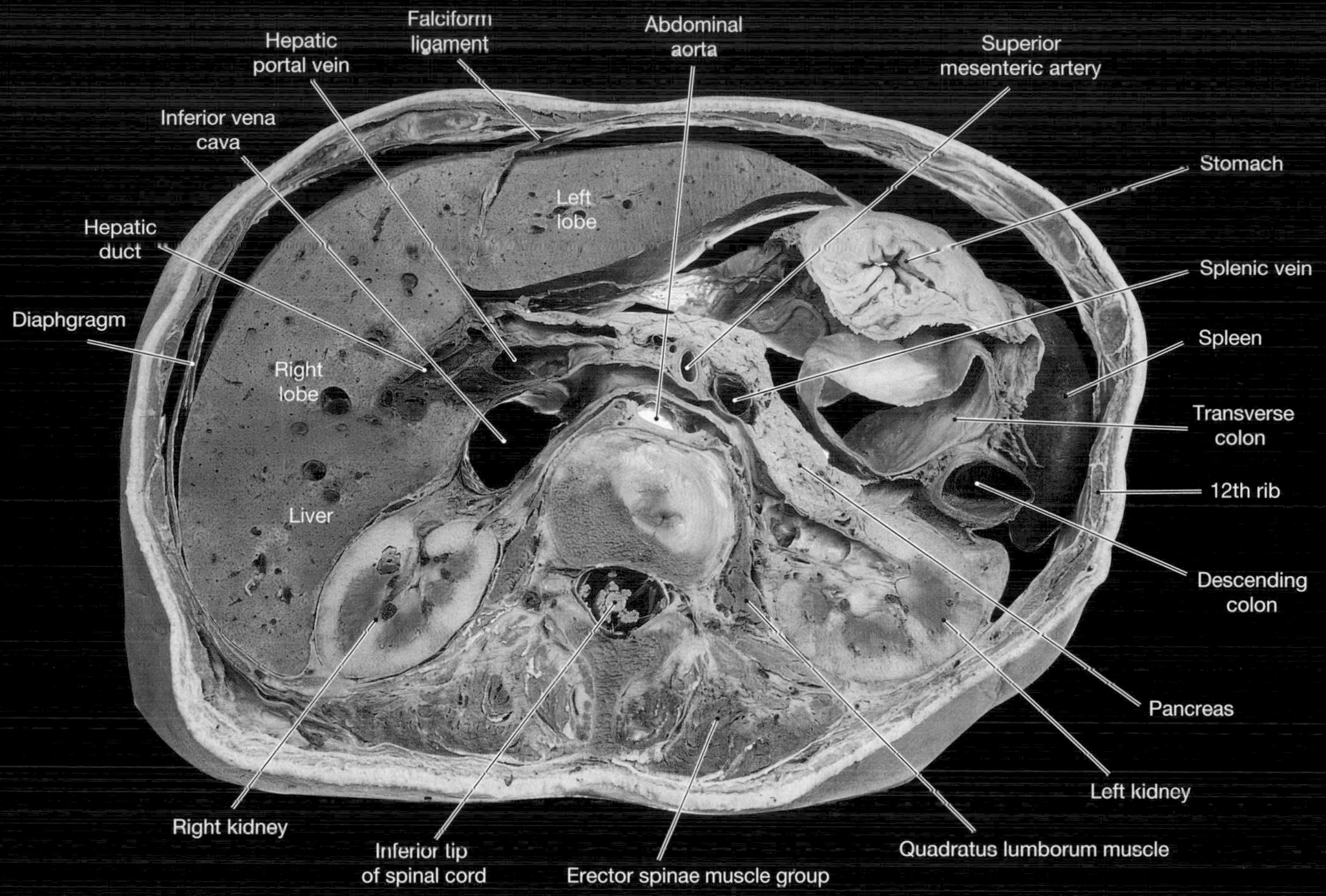

Hepatic portal vein
Falciform ligament
Abdominal aorta
Superior mesenteric artery
Inferior vena cava
Left lobe
Stomach
Hepatic duct
Splenic vein
Diaphgragm
Spleen
Right lobe
Transverse colon
Liver
12th rib
Descending colon
Pancreas
Left kidney
Right kidney
Inferior tip of spinal cord
Erector spinae muscle group
Quadratus lumborum muscle

PLATE **57a** ABDOMINAL CAVITY, HORIZONTAL SECTION AT T_{12}

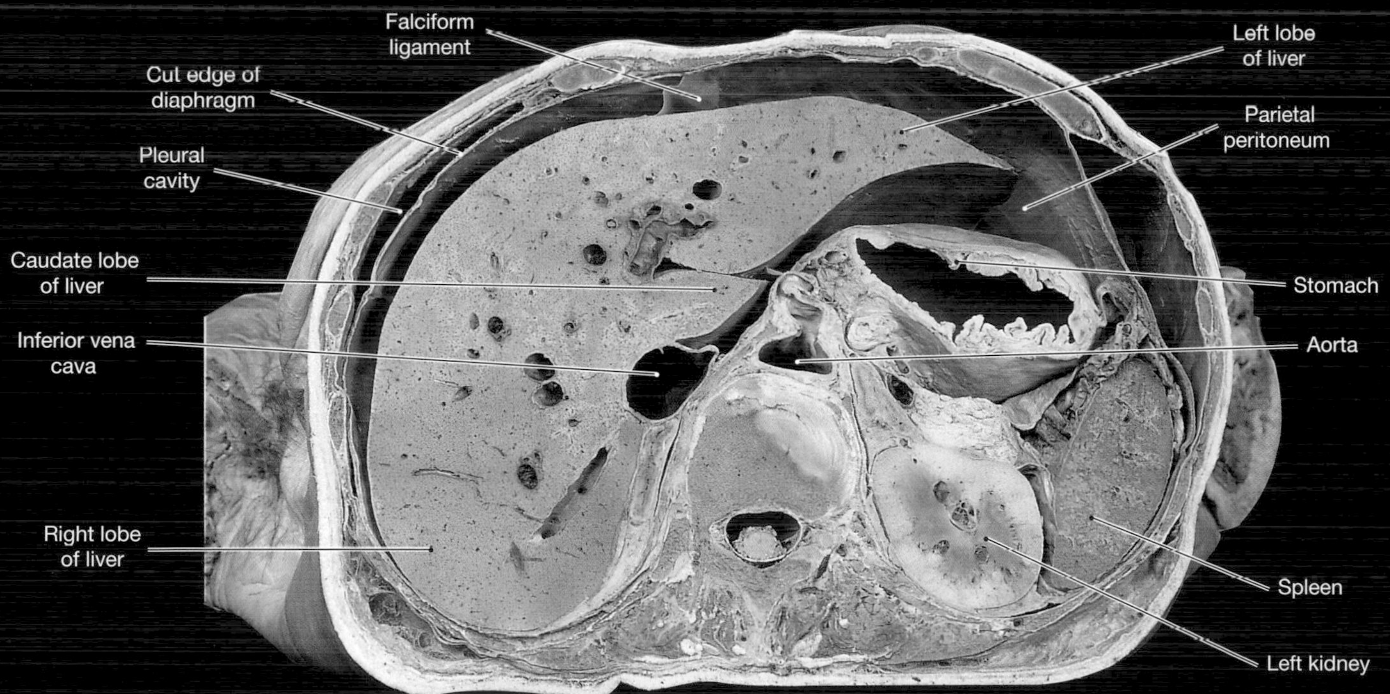

Falciform ligament
Left lobe of liver
Cut edge of diaphragm
Parietal peritoneum
Pleural cavity
Caudate lobe of liver
Stomach
Inferior vena cava
Aorta
Right lobe of liver
Spleen
Left kidney

PLATE **57b** ABDOMINAL CAVITY, HORIZONTAL SECTION AT L_1

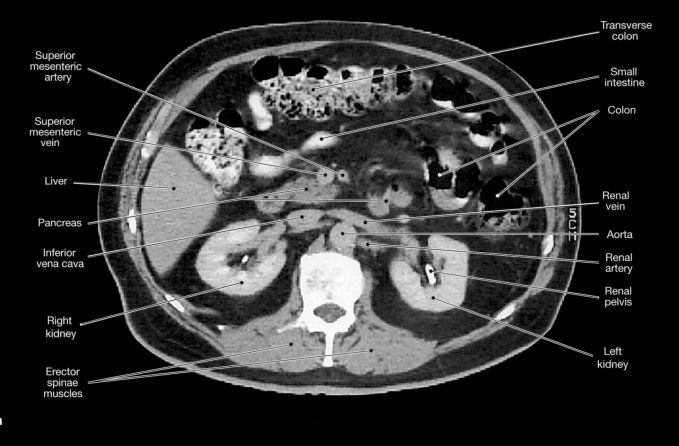

Superior mesenteric artery

Superior mesenteric vein

Liver

Pancreas

Inferior vena cava

Right kidney

Erector spinae muscles

Transverse colon

Small intestine

Colon

Renal vein

Aorta

Renal artery

Renal pelvis

Left kidney

5 C M

58a

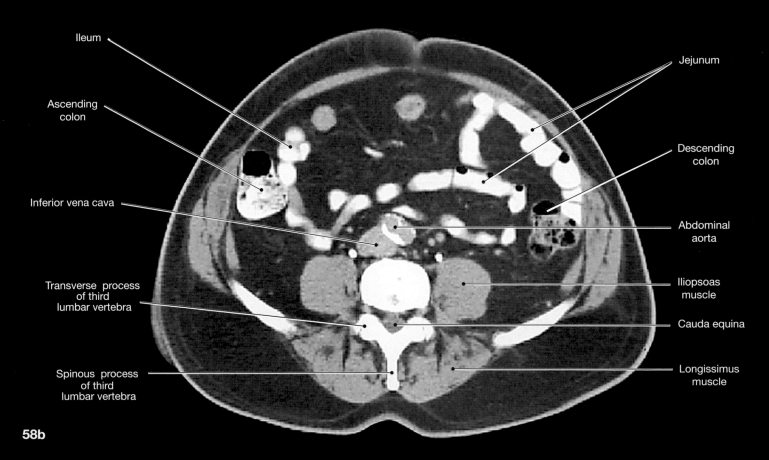

Ileum

Ascending colon

Inferior vena cava

Transverse process of third lumbar vertebra

Spinous process of third lumbar vertebra

Jejunum

Descending colon

Abdominal aorta

Iliopsoas muscle

Cauda equina

Longissimus muscle

58b

PLATES 58a–b MRI SCANS OF THE TRUNK, HORIZONTAL SECTIONS, SUPERIOR TO INFERIOR SEQUENCE

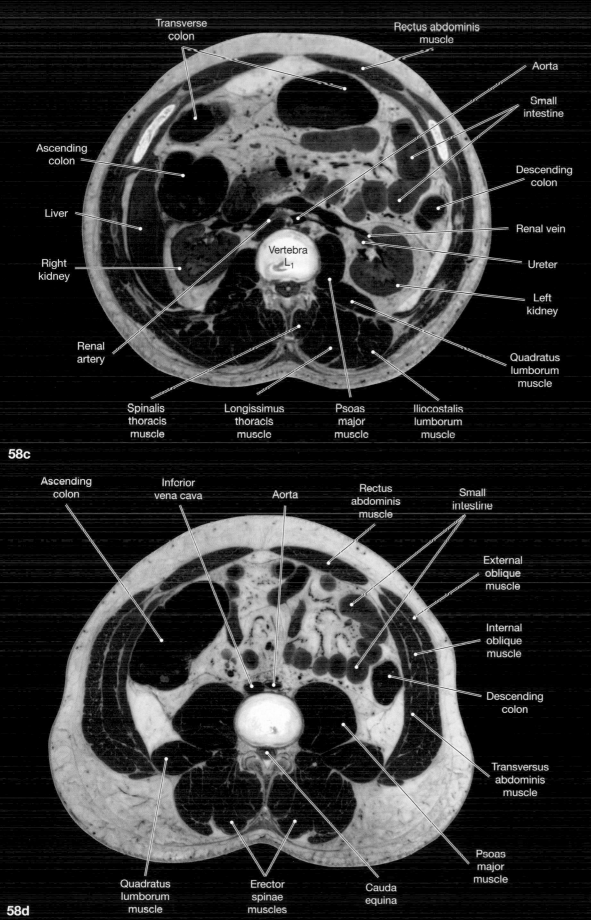

Transverse colon

Rectus abdominis muscle

Aorta

Small intestine

Ascending colon

Descending colon

Liver

Renal vein

Right kidney

Vertebra L₁

Ureter

Left kidney

Renal artery

Quadratus lumborum muscle

Spinalis thoracis muscle

Longissimus thoracis muscle

Psoas major muscle

Iliocostalis lumborum muscle

58c

Ascending colon

Inferior vena cava

Aorta

Rectus abdominis muscle

Small intestine

External oblique muscle

Internal oblique muscle

Descending colon

Transversus abdominis muscle

Psoas major muscle

Quadratus lumborum muscle

Erector spinae muscles

Cauda equina

58d

PLATES 58c–d
HORIZONTAL SECTIONS
THROUGH THE TRUNK

These sections, derived from the Visible Human dataset, are at the approximate levels of the scans shown in part a–b.

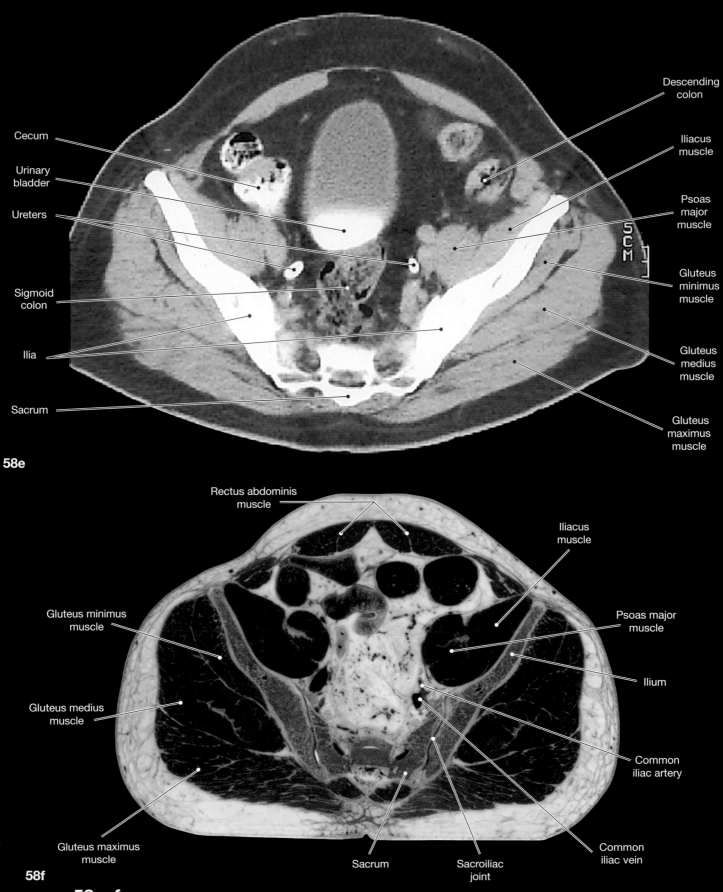

Cecum

Urinary bladder

Ureters

Sigmoid colon

Ilia

Sacrum

Descending colon

Iliacus muscle

Psoas major muscle

Gluteus minimus muscle

Gluteus medius muscle

Gluteus maximus muscle

58e

Rectus abdominis muscle

Iliacus muscle

Gluteus minimus muscle

Psoas major muscle

Gluteus medius muscle

Ilium

Common iliac artery

Gluteus maximus muscle

Sacrum

Sacroiliac joint

Common iliac vein

58f

PLATES 58e–f HORIZONTAL SECTIONS THROUGH THE TRUNK.

Part f, derived from the Visible Human dataset, is at the approximate level of the MRI scan in part e.

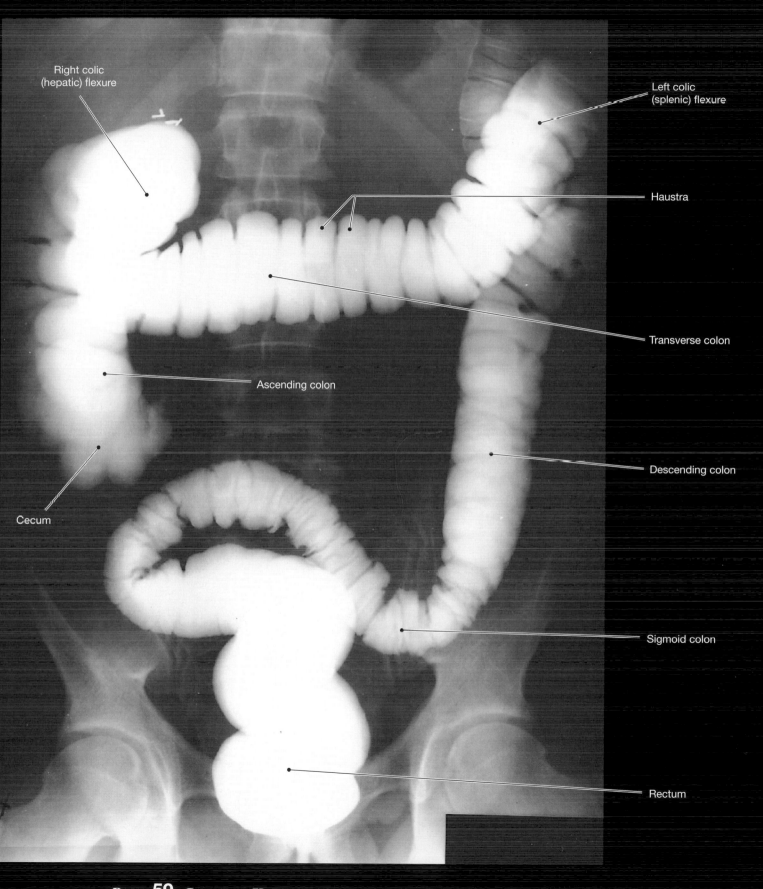

Right colic
(hepatic) flexure

Left colic
(splenic) flexure

Haustra

Transverse colon

Ascending colon

Descending colon

Cecum

Sigmoid colon

Rectum

PLATE **59** CONTRAST X-RAY OF COLON AND RECTUM, ANTERIOR-POSTERIOR PROJECTION

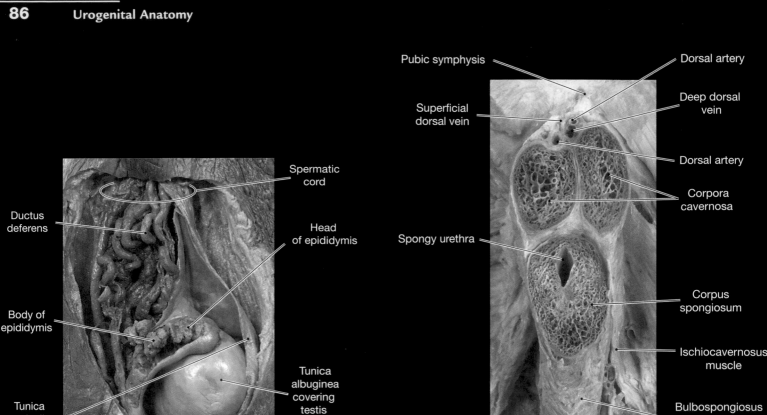

Spermatic
cord

Ductus
deferens

Head
of epididymis

Body of
epididymis

Tunica
albuginea
covering
testis

Tunica
vaginalis
(reflected)

Tail
of epididymis

PLATE 60a   **TESTIS AND EPIDIDYMIS**

Pubic symphysis

Dorsal artery

Superficial
dorsal vein

Deep dorsal
vein

Dorsal artery

Corpora
cavernosa

Spongy urethra

Corpus
spongiosum

Ischiocavernosus
muscle

Bulbospongiosus
muscle overlying
shaft of penis

PLATE 60b   **CROSS SECTION THROUGH DISSECTED PENIS**

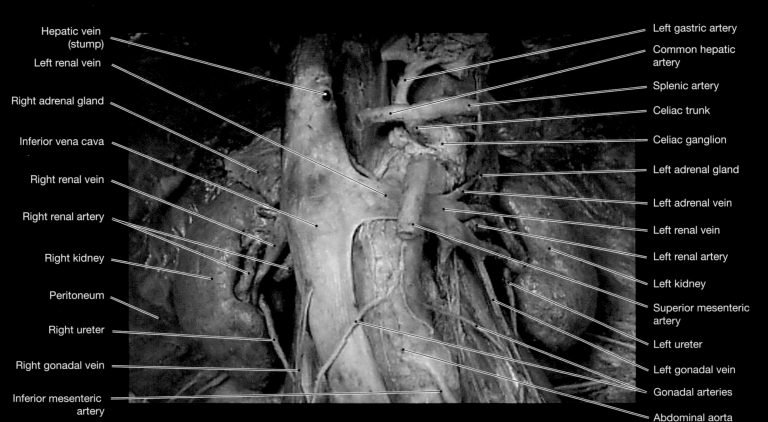

Hepatic vein
(stump)

Left renal vein

Right adrenal gland

Inferior vena cava

Right renal vein

Right renal artery

Right kidney

Peritoneum

Right ureter

Right gonadal vein

Inferior mesenteric
artery

Left gastric artery

Common hepatic
artery

Splenic artery

Celiac trunk

Celiac ganglion

Left adrenal gland

Left adrenal vein

Left renal vein

Left renal artery

Left kidney

Superior mesenteric
artery

Left ureter

Left gonadal vein

Gonadal arteries

Abdominal aorta

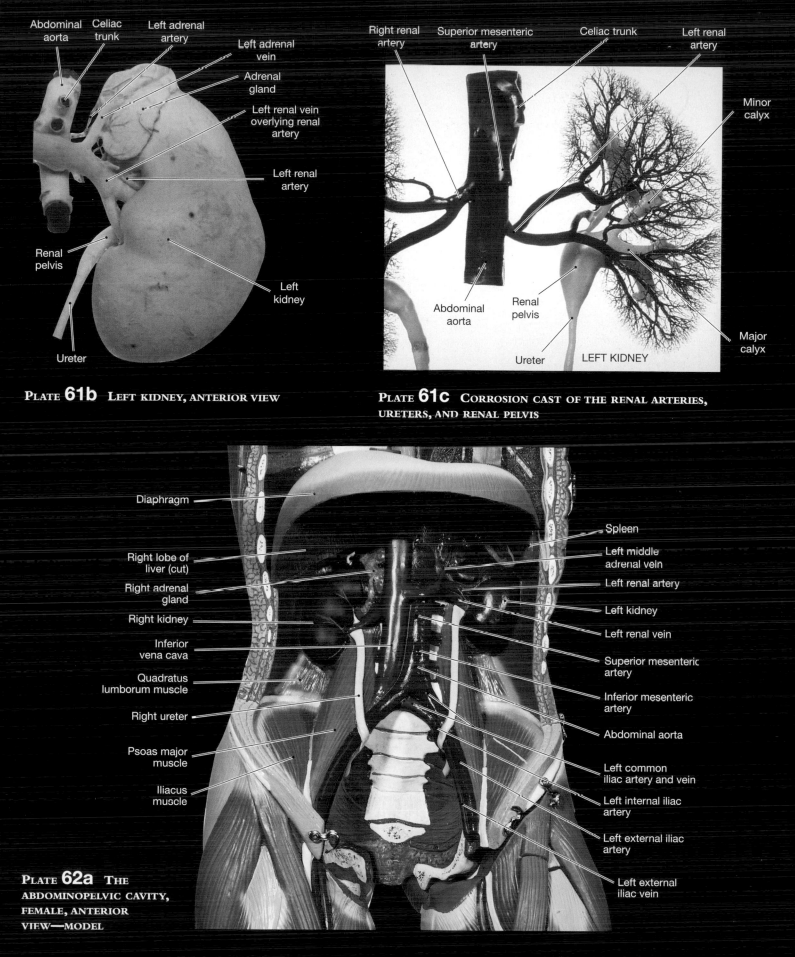

Plate 61b Left kidney, anterior view

Abdominal aorta
Celiac trunk
Left adrenal artery
Left adrenal vein
Adrenal gland
Left renal vein overlying renal artery
Left renal artery
Renal pelvis
Left kidney
Ureter

Plate 61c Corrosion cast of the renal arteries, ureters, and renal pelvis

Right renal artery
Superior mesenteric artery
Celiac trunk
Left renal artery
Minor calyx
Abdominal aorta
Renal pelvis
Ureter
LEFT KIDNEY
Major calyx

Plate 62a The abdominopelvic cavity, female, anterior view—model

Diaphragm
Right lobe of liver (cut)
Right adrenal gland
Right kidney
Inferior vena cava
Quadratus lumborum muscle
Right ureter
Psoas major muscle
Iliacus muscle

Spleen
Left middle adrenal vein
Left renal artery
Left kidney
Left renal vein
Superior mesenteric artery
Inferior mesenteric artery
Abdominal aorta
Left common iliac artery and vein
Left internal iliac artery
Left external iliac artery
Left external iliac vein

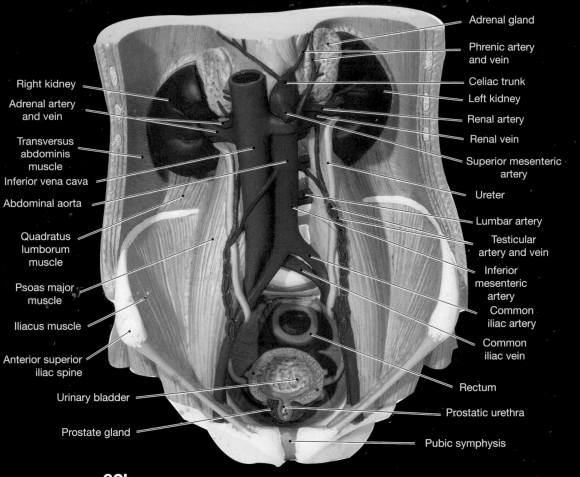

Adrenal gland

Phrenic artery
and vein

Right kidney

Adrenal artery
and vein

Transversus
abdominis
muscle

Inferior vena cava

Abdominal aorta

Quadratus
lumborum
muscle

Psoas major
muscle

Iliacus muscle

Anterior superior
iliac spine

Urinary bladder

Prostate gland

Celiac trunk

Left kidney

Renal artery

Renal vein

Superior mesenteric
artery

Ureter

Lumbar artery

Testicular
artery and vein

Inferior
mesenteric
artery

Common
iliac artery

Common
iliac vein

Rectum

Prostatic urethra

Pubic symphysis

PLATE **62b** THE ABDOMINOPELVIC CAVITY, MALE, ANTERIOR VIEW—MODEL

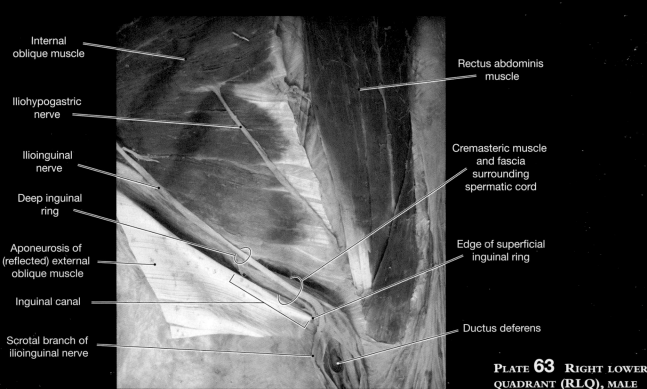

Internal
oblique muscle

Iliohypogastric
nerve

Ilioinguinal
nerve

Deep inguinal
ring

Aponeurosis of
(reflected) external
oblique muscle

Inguinal canal

Scrotal branch of
ilioinguinal nerve

Rectus abdominis
muscle

Cremasteric muscle
and fascia
surrounding
spermatic cord

Edge of superficial
inguinal ring

Ductus deferens

PLATE **63** RIGHT LOWER
QUADRANT (RLQ), MALE

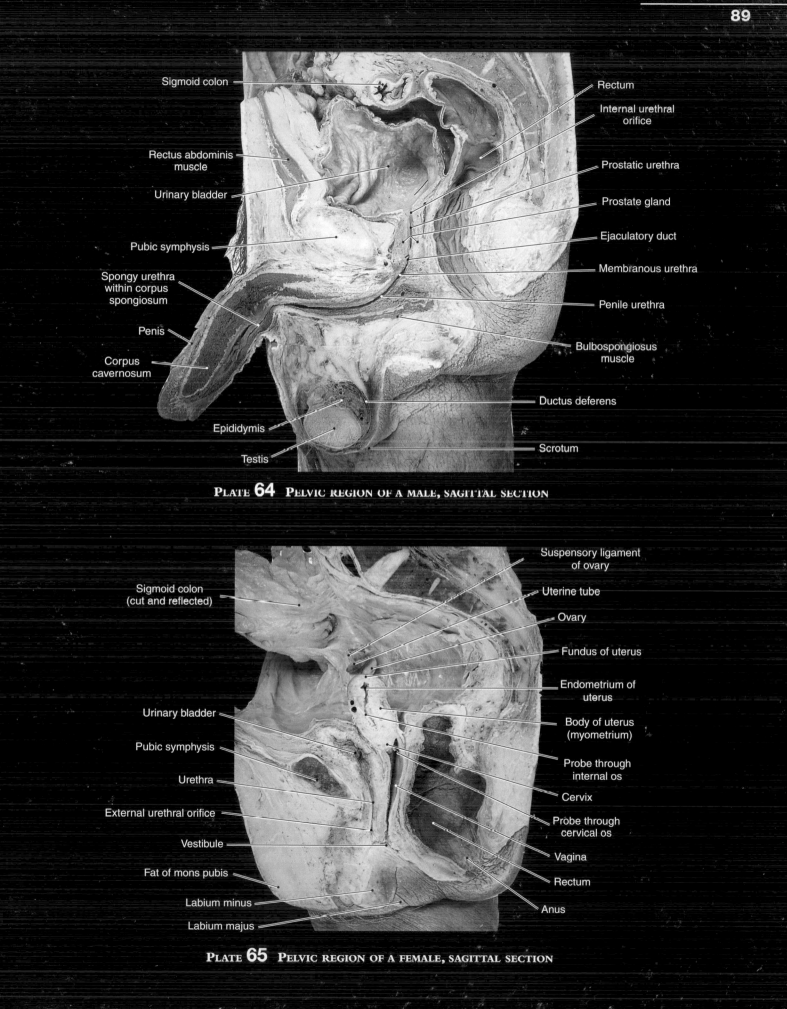

Sigmoid colon

Rectus abdominis muscle

Urinary bladder

Pubic symphysis

Spongy urethra within corpus spongiosum

Penis

Corpus cavernosum

Epididymis

Testis

Rectum

Internal urethral orifice

Prostatic urethra

Prostate gland

Ejaculatory duct

Membranous urethra

Penile urethra

Bulbospongiosus muscle

Ductus deferens

Scrotum

PLATE 64 PELVIC REGION OF A MALE, SAGITTAL SECTION

Sigmoid colon (cut and reflected)

Urinary bladder

Pubic symphysis

Urethra

External urethral orifice

Vestibule

Fat of mons pubis

Labium minus

Labium majus

Suspensory ligament of ovary

Uterine tube

Ovary

Fundus of uterus

Endometrium of uterus

Body of uterus (myometrium)

Probe through internal os

Cervix

Probe through cervical os

Vagina

Rectum

Anus

PLATE 65 PELVIC REGION OF A FEMALE, SAGITTAL SECTION

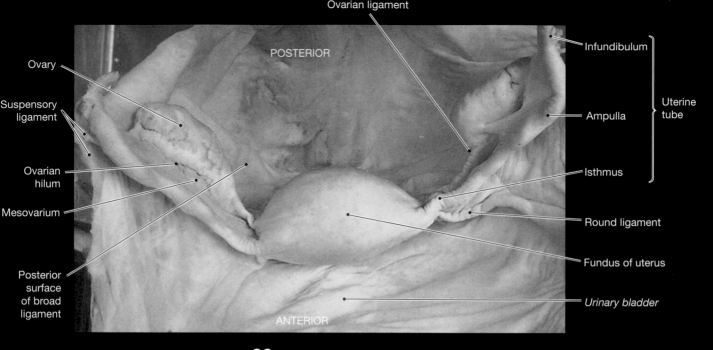

Ovarian ligament

POSTERIOR

Infundibulum

Ovary

Suspensory
ligament

Ampulla

Uterine
tube

Ovarian
hilum

Isthmus

Mesovarium

Round ligament

Fundus of uterus

Posterior
surface
of broad
ligament

ANTERIOR

Urinary bladder

PLATE **66** PELVIC CAVITY, SUPERIOR VIEW

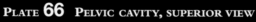

Uterine tubes

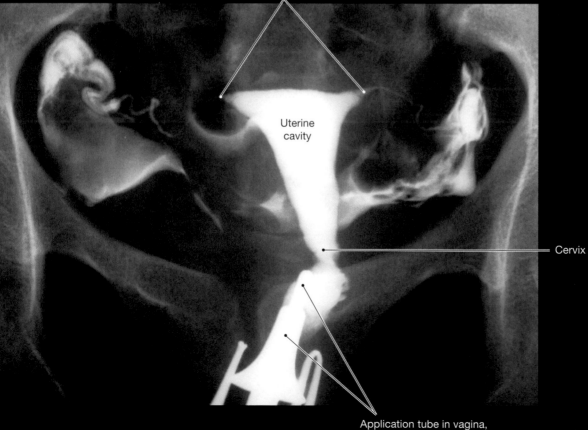

Uterine
cavity

Cervix

Application tube in vagina,
source of contrast medium

PLATE **67** HYSTEROSALPINGOGRAM

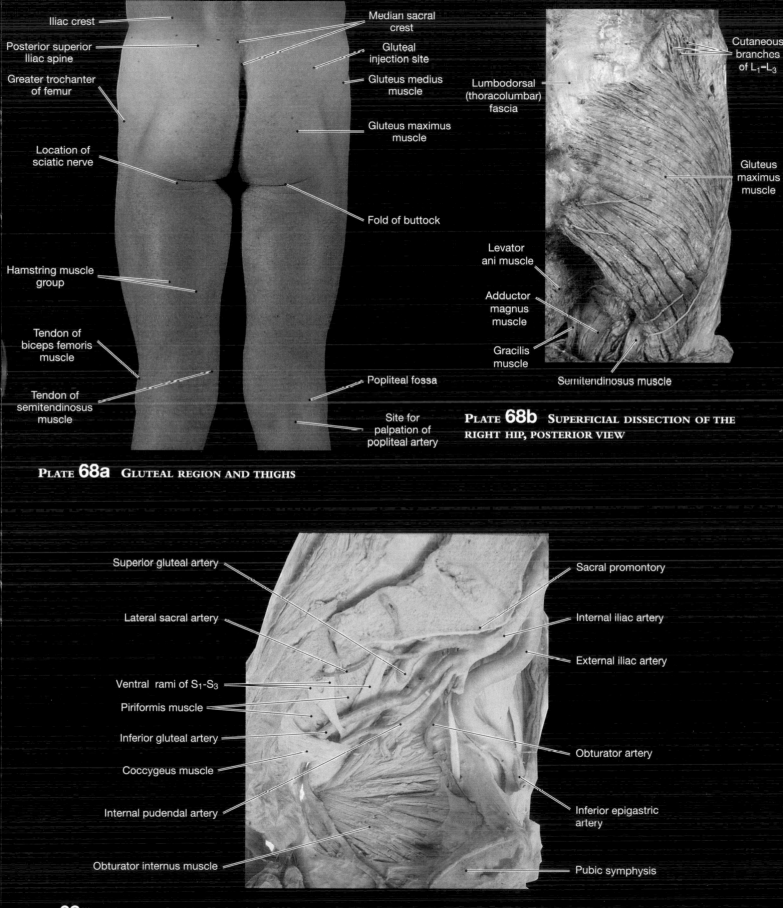

Iliac crest

Posterior superior
Iliac spine

Greater trochanter
of femur

Location of
sciatic nerve

Hamstring muscle
group

Tendon of
biceps femoris
muscle

Tendon of
semitendinosus
muscle

Median sacral
crest

Gluteal
injection site

Gluteus medius
muscle

Gluteus maximus
muscle

Fold of buttock

Popliteal fossa

Site for
palpation of
popliteal artery

PLATE 68a GLUTEAL REGION AND THIGHS

Cutaneous
branches
of L₁–L₃

Lumbodorsal
(thoracolumbar)
fascia

Gluteus
maximus
muscle

Levator
ani muscle

Adductor
magnus
muscle

Gracilis
muscle

Semitendinosus muscle

**PLATE 68b SUPERFICIAL DISSECTION OF THE
RIGHT HIP, POSTERIOR VIEW**

Superior gluteal artery

Lateral sacral artery

Ventral rami of S₁-S₃

Piriformis muscle

Inferior gluteal artery

Coccygeus muscle

Internal pudendal artery

Obturator internus muscle

Sacral promontory

Internal iliac artery

External iliac artery

Obturator artery

Inferior epigastric
artery

Pubic symphysis

PLATE 68c BLOOD VESSELS, NERVES, AND MUSCLES IN THE LEFT HALF OF THE PELVIS

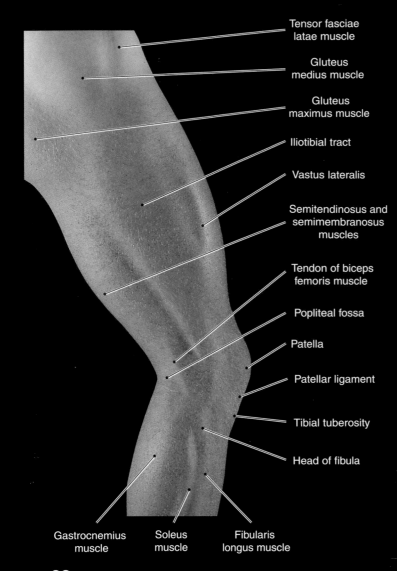

Tensor fasciae
latae muscle

Gluteus
medius muscle

Gluteus
maximus muscle

Iliotibial tract

Vastus lateralis

Semitendinosus and
semimembranosus
muscles

Tendon of biceps
femoris muscle

Popliteal fossa

Patella

Patellar ligament

Tibial tuberosity

Head of fibula

Gastrocnemius
muscle

Soleus
muscle

Fibularis
longus muscle

PLATE 69a **SURFACE ANATOMY OF THE THIGH,**
LATERAL VIEW

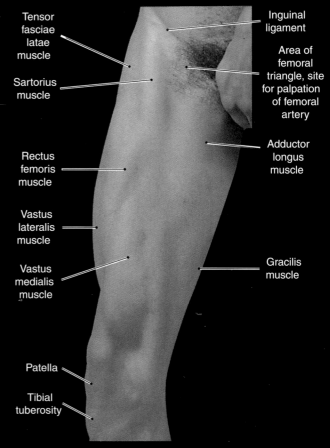

Tensor
fasciae
latae
muscle

Sartorius
muscle

Rectus
femoris
muscle

Vastus
lateralis
muscle

Vastus
medialis
muscle

Patella

Tibial
tuberosity

Inguinal
ligament

Area of
femoral
triangle, site
for palpation
of femoral
artery

Adductor
longus
muscle

Gracilis
muscle

PLATE 69b **SURFACE ANATOMY OF RIGHT THIGH,**

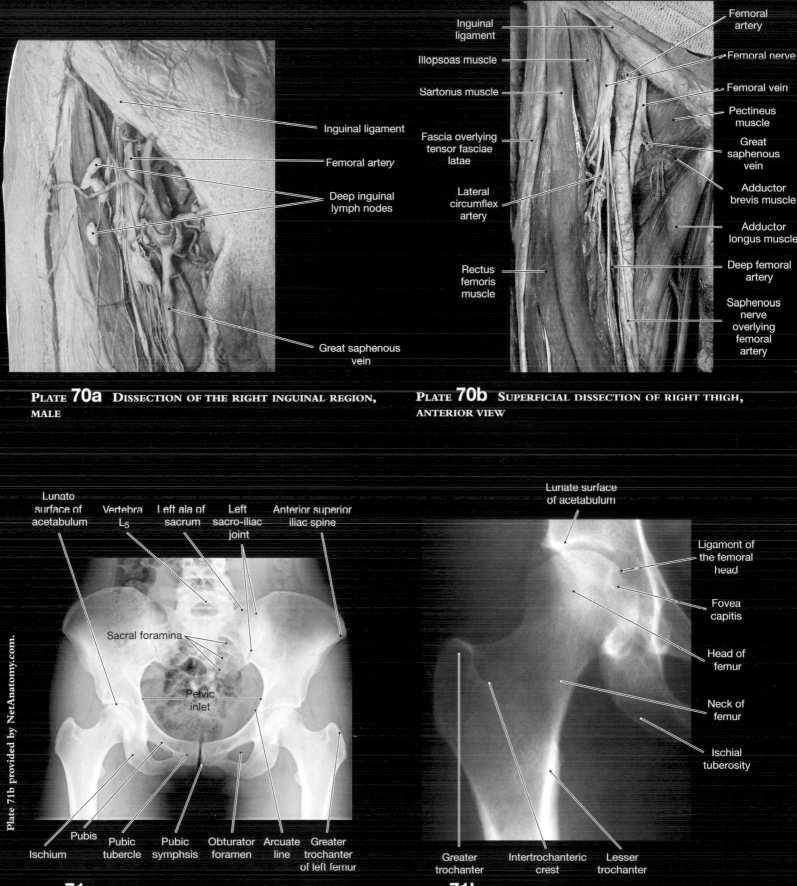

Inguinal ligament

Femoral artery

Deep inguinal
lymph nodes

Great saphenous
vein

Inguinal
ligament

Iliopsoas muscle

Sartorius muscle

Fascia overlying
tensor fasciae
latae

Lateral
circumflex
artery

Rectus
femoris
muscle

Femoral
artery

Femoral nerve

Femoral vein

Pectineus
muscle

Great
saphenous
vein

Adductor
brevis muscle

Adductor
longus muscle

Deep femoral
artery

Saphenous
nerve
overlying
femoral
artery

PLATE 70a DISSECTION OF THE RIGHT INGUINAL REGION,
MALE

PLATE 70b SUPERFICIAL DISSECTION OF RIGHT THIGH,
ANTERIOR VIEW

Lunate
surface of
acetabulum

Vertebra
L5

Left ala of
sacrum

Left
sacro-iliac
joint

Anterior superior
iliac spine

Sacral foramina

Pelvic
inlet

Ischium

Pubis

Pubic
tubercle

Pubic
symphsis

Obturator
foramen

Arcuate
line

Greater
trochanter
of left femur

Lunate surface
of acetabulum

Ligament of
the femoral
head

Fovea
capitis

Head of
femur

Neck of
femur

Ischial
tuberosity

Greater
trochanter

Intertrochanteric
crest

Lesser
trochanter

PLATE 71a X-RAY OF PELVIS AND PROXIMAL FEMORA,
ANTERIOR-POSTERIOR PROJECTION

PLATE 71b X-RAY OF THE RIGHT HIP JOINT, ANTERIOR-
POSTERIOR PROJECTION

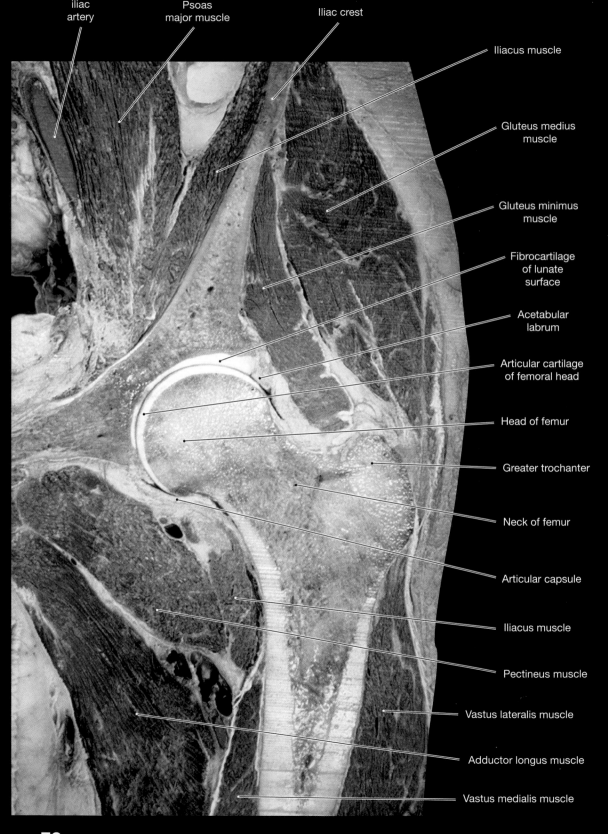

iliac artery

Psoas major muscle

Iliac crest

Iliacus muscle

Gluteus medius muscle

Gluteus minimus muscle

Fibrocartilage of lunate surface

Acetabular labrum

Articular cartilage of femoral head

Head of femur

Greater trochanter

Neck of femur

Articular capsule

Iliacus muscle

Pectineus muscle

Vastus lateralis muscle

Adductor longus muscle

Vastus medialis muscle

PLATE **72a** CORONAL SECTION THROUGH THE LEFT HIP

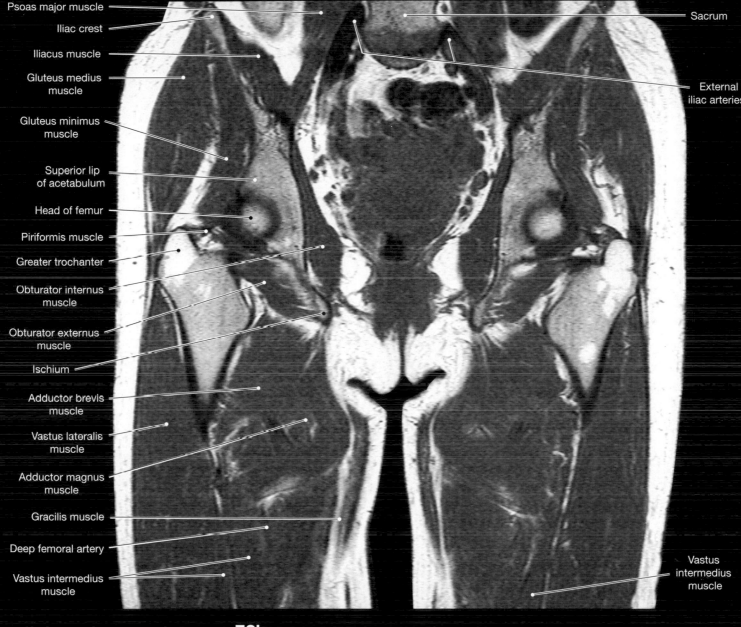

Psoas major muscle

Iliac crest

Iliacus muscle

Gluteus medius
muscle

Gluteus minimus
muscle

Superior lip
of acetabulum

Head of femur

Piriformis muscle

Greater trochanter

Obturator internus
muscle

Obturator externus
muscle

Ischium

Adductor brevis
muscle

Vastus lateralis
muscle

Adductor magnus
muscle

Gracilis muscle

Deep femoral artery

Vastus intermedius
muscle

Sacrum

External
iliac arteries

Vastus
intermedius
muscle

PLATE **72b** MRI SCAN OF PELVIC REGION, FRONTAL SECTION

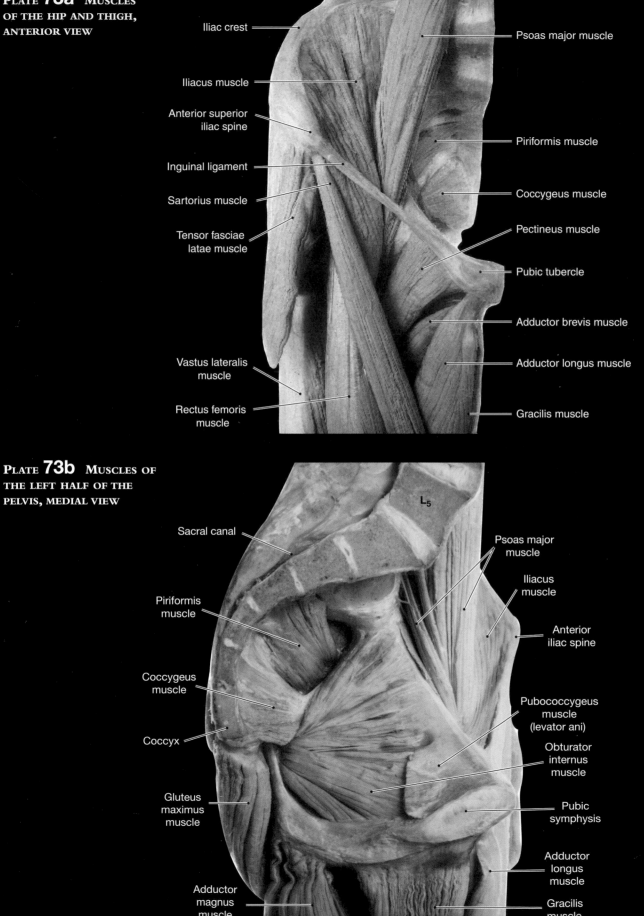

PLATE 73a MUSCLES OF THE HIP AND THIGH, ANTERIOR VIEW

Iliac crest

Iliacus muscle

Anterior superior iliac spine

Inguinal ligament

Sartorius muscle

Tensor fasciae latae muscle

Vastus lateralis muscle

Rectus femoris muscle

Psoas major muscle

Piriformis muscle

Coccygeus muscle

Pectineus muscle

Pubic tubercle

Adductor brevis muscle

Adductor longus muscle

Gracilis muscle

PLATE 73b MUSCLES OF THE LEFT HALF OF THE PELVIS, MEDIAL VIEW

L₅

Sacral canal

Piriformis muscle

Coccygeus muscle

Coccyx

Gluteus maximus muscle

Adductor magnus muscle

Psoas major muscle

Iliacus muscle

Anterior iliac spine

Pubococcygeus muscle (levator ani)

Obturator internus muscle

Pubic symphysis

Adductor longus muscle

Gracilis muscle

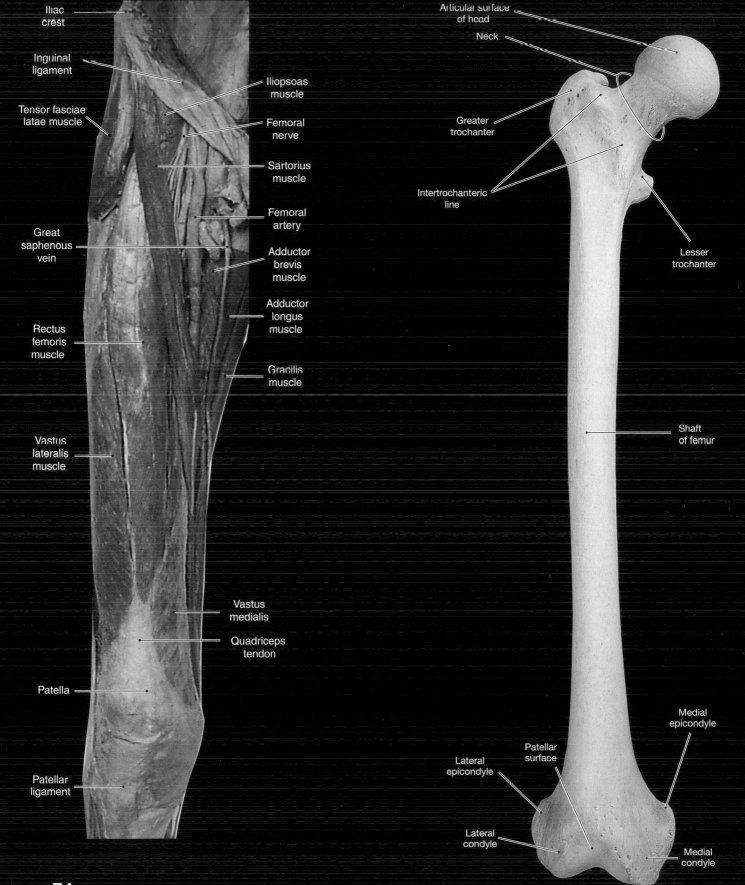

Iliac crest

Inguinal ligament

Tensor fasciae latae muscle

Great saphenous vein

Rectus femoris muscle

Vastus lateralis muscle

Patella

Patellar ligament

Iliopsoas muscle

Femoral nerve

Sartorius muscle

Femoral artery

Adductor brevis muscle

Adductor longus muscle

Gracilis muscle

Vastus medialis

Quadriceps tendon

Articular surface of head

Neck

Greater trochanter

Intertrochanteric line

Lesser trochanter

Shaft of femur

Medial epicondyle

Patellar surface

Lateral epicondyle

Lateral condyle

Medial condyle

PLATE **74** SUPERFICIAL DISSECTION OF RIGHT LOWER
LIMB, ANTERIOR VIEW

PLATE **75a** RIGHT FEMUR, ANTERIOR VIEW

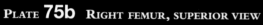

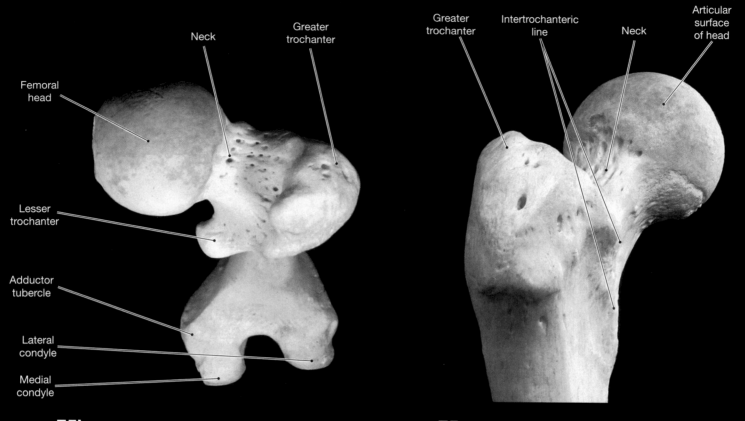

Neck

Greater trochanter

Femoral head

Lesser trochanter

Adductor tubercle

Lateral condyle

Medial condyle

PLATE 75b RIGHT FEMUR, SUPERIOR VIEW

Greater trochanter

Intertrochanteric line

Neck

Articular surface of head

PLATE 75c HEAD OF RIGHT FEMUR, LATERAL VIEW

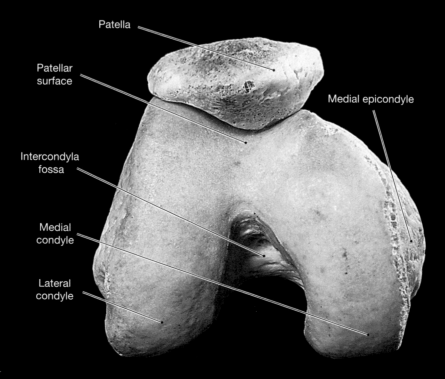

Patella

Patellar surface

Medial epicondyle

Intercondyla fossa

Medial condyle

Lateral condyle

PLATE 75d RIGHT FEMUR, INFERIOR VIEW

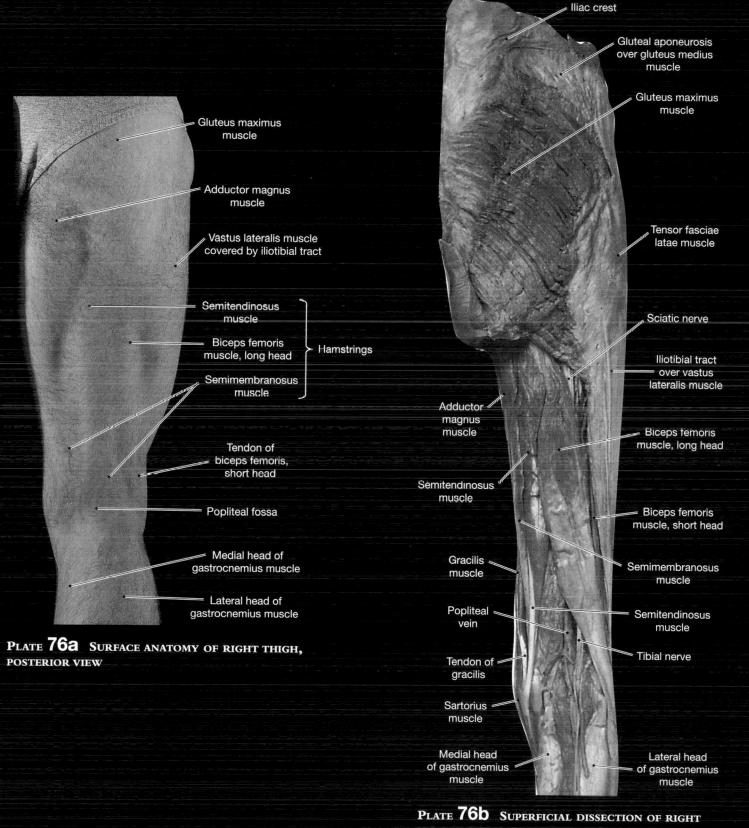

Iliac crest

Gluteal aponeurosis
over gluteus medius
muscle

Gluteus maximus
muscle

Gluteus maximus
muscle

Adductor magnus
muscle

Tensor fasciae
latae muscle

Vastus lateralis muscle
covered by iliotibial tract

Semitendinosus
muscle

Sciatic nerve

Biceps femoris
muscle, long head

Hamstrings

Iliotibial tract
over vastus
lateralis muscle

Semimembranosus
muscle

Adductor
magnus
muscle

Biceps femoris
muscle, long head

Tendon of
biceps femoris,
short head

Semitendinosus
muscle

Biceps femoris
muscle, short head

Popliteal fossa

Gracilis
muscle

Semimembranosus
muscle

Medial head of
gastrocnemius muscle

Popliteal
vein

Semitendinosus
muscle

Lateral head of
gastrocnemius muscle

Tibial nerve

Tendon of
gracilis

PLATE 76a SURFACE ANATOMY OF RIGHT THIGH,
POSTERIOR VIEW

Sartorius
muscle

Medial head
of gastrocnemius
muscle

Lateral head
of gastrocnemius
muscle

PLATE 76b SUPERFICIAL DISSECTION OF RIGHT
HIP AND THIGH, POSTERIOR VIEW

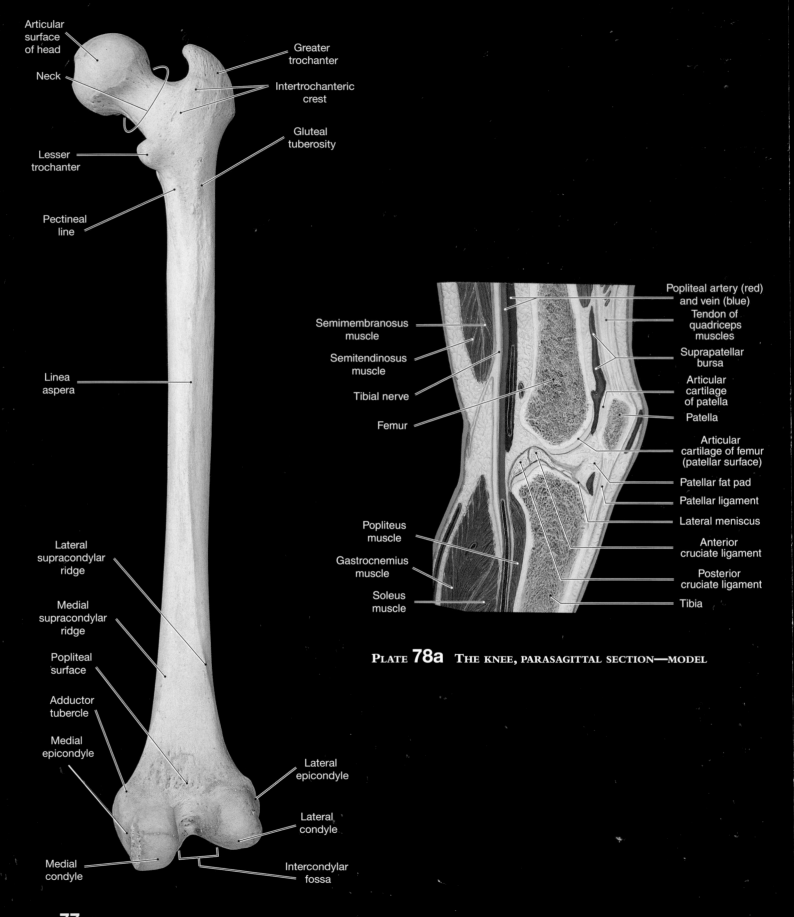

Articular surface of head

Neck

Lesser trochanter

Pectineal line

Greater trochanter

Intertrochanteric crest

Gluteal tuberosity

Linea aspera

Lateral supracondylar ridge

Medial supracondylar ridge

Popliteal surface

Adductor tubercle

Medial epicondyle

Lateral epicondyle

Lateral condyle

Medial condyle

Intercondylar fossa

Semimembranosus muscle

Semitendinosus muscle

Tibial nerve

Femur

Popliteus muscle

Gastrocnemius muscle

Soleus muscle

Popliteal artery (red) and vein (blue)

Tendon of quadriceps muscles

Suprapatellar bursa

Articular cartilage of patella

Patella

Articular cartilage of femur (patellar surface)

Patellar fat pad

Patellar ligament

Lateral meniscus

Anterior cruciate ligament

Posterior cruciate ligament

Tibia

PLATE 78a   THE KNEE, PARASAGITTAL SECTION—MODEL

PLATE 77   RIGHT FEMUR, POSTERIOR VIEW

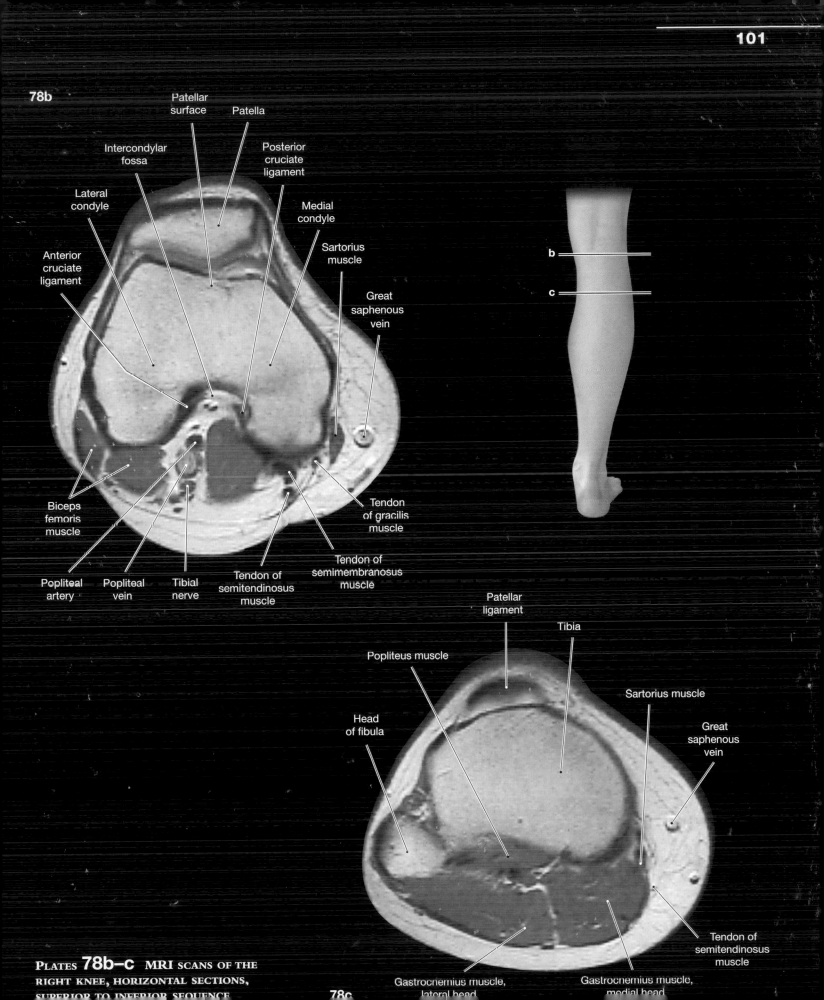

78b

Patellar surface

Patella

Intercondylar fossa

Posterior cruciate ligament

Lateral condyle

Medial condyle

Anterior cruciate ligament

Sartorius muscle

Great saphenous vein

Biceps femoris muscle

Tendon of gracilis muscle

Tendon of semimembranosus muscle

Popliteal artery

Popliteal vein

Tibial nerve

Tendon of semitendinosus muscle

b

c

Patellar ligament

Tibia

Popliteus muscle

Sartorius muscle

Head of fibula

Great saphenous vein

Tendon of semitendinosus muscle

Gastrocnemius muscle, lateral head

Gastrocnemius muscle, medial head

PLATES 78b–c MRI SCANS OF THE RIGHT KNEE, HORIZONTAL SECTIONS, SUPERIOR TO INFERIOR SEQUENCE

78c

78d

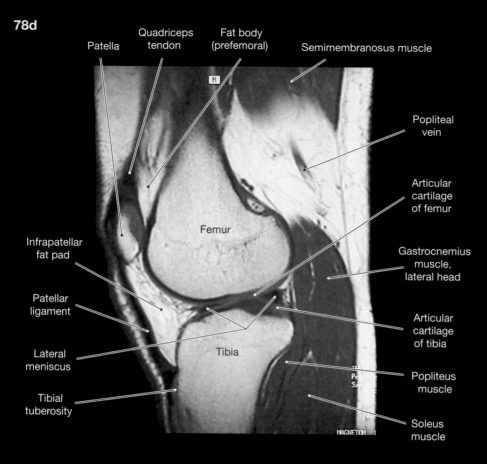

Patella

Quadriceps tendon

Fat body (prefemoral)

Semimembranosus muscle

Popliteal vein

Articular cartilage of femur

Gastrocnemius muscle, lateral head

Articular cartilage of tibia

Popliteus muscle

Soleus muscle

Infrapatellar fat pad

Patellar ligament

Lateral meniscus

Tibial tuberosity

Femur

Tibia

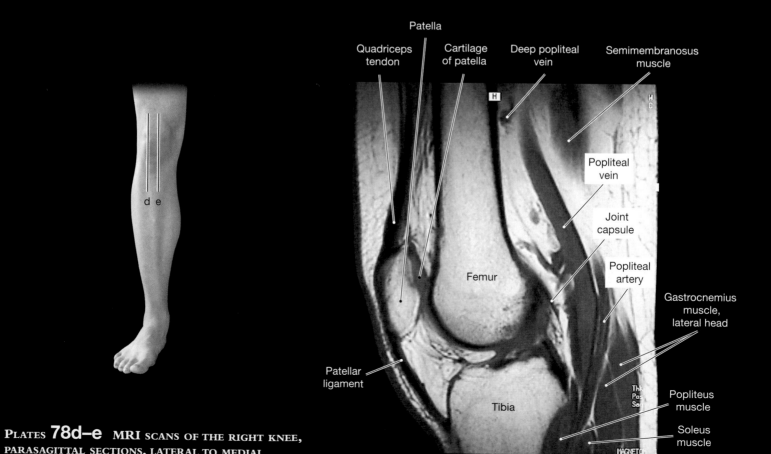

d e

Patella

Quadriceps tendon

Cartilage of patella

Deep popliteal vein

Semimembranosus muscle

Popliteal vein

Joint capsule

Popliteal artery

Gastrocnemius muscle, lateral head

Popliteus muscle

Soleus muscle

Patellar ligament

Femur

Tibia

PLATES **78d–e** MRI SCANS OF THE RIGHT KNEE, PARASAGITTAL SECTIONS, LATERAL TO MEDIAL

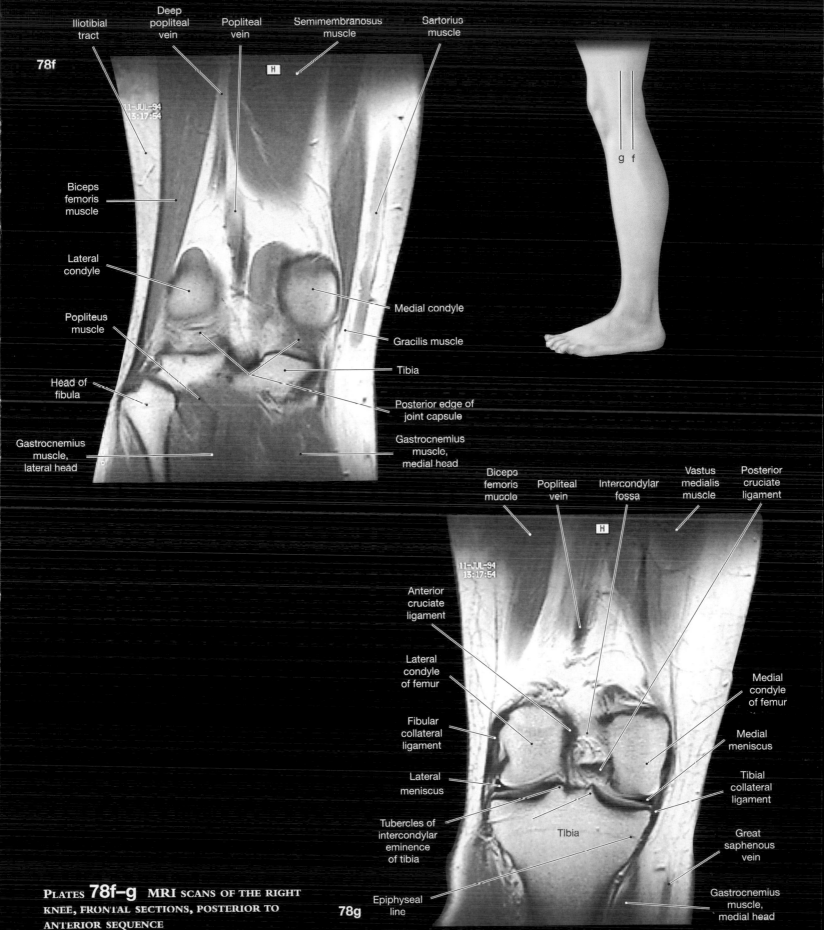

Iliotibial tract

Deep popliteal vein

Popliteal vein

Semimembranosus muscle

Sartorius muscle

78f

Biceps femoris muscle

Lateral condyle

Medial condyle

Popliteus muscle

Gracilis muscle

Tibia

Head of fibula

Posterior edge of joint capsule

Gastrocnemius muscle, lateral head

Gastrocnemius muscle, medial head

g f

Biceps femoris muscle

Popliteal vein

Intercondylar fossa

Vastus medialis muscle

Posterior cruciate ligament

Anterior cruciate ligament

Lateral condyle of femur

Medial condyle of femur

Fibular collateral ligament

Medial meniscus

Lateral meniscus

Tibial collateral ligament

Tubercles of intercondylar eminence of tibia

Tibia

Great saphenous vein

Epiphyseal line

78g

Gastrocnemius muscle, medial head

PLATES 78f–g MRI SCANS OF THE RIGHT KNEE, FRONTAL SECTIONS, POSTERIOR TO ANTERIOR SEQUENCE

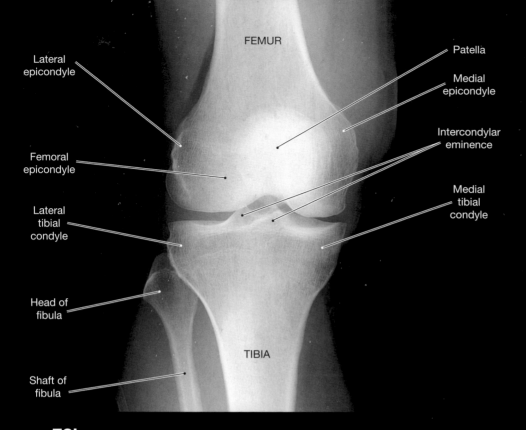

Lateral
epicondyle

FEMUR

Patella

Medial
epicondyle

Femoral
epicondyle

Intercondylar
eminence

Lateral
tibial
condyle

Medial
tibial
condyle

Head of
fibula

TIBIA

Shaft of
fibula

PLATE 78h X-RAY OF THE EXTENDED RIGHT KNEE, ANTERIOR–POSTERIOR PROJECTION

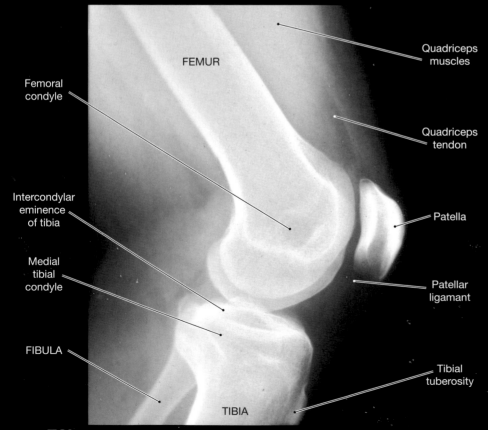

FEMUR

Quadriceps
muscles

Femoral
condyle

Quadriceps
tendon

Intercondylar
eminence
of tibia

Patella

Medial
tibial
condyle

Patellar
ligamant

FIBULA

Tibial
tuberosity

TIBIA

PLATE 78i X-RAY OF THE PARTIALLY FLEXED RIGHT KNEE, LATERAL PROJECTION

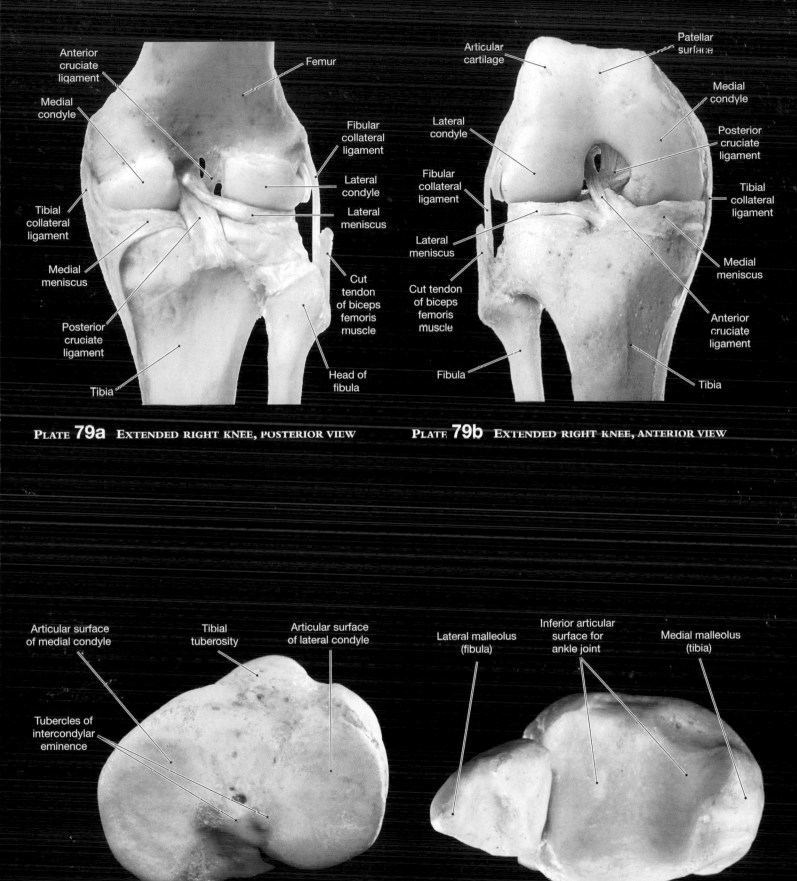

PLATE 79a EXTENDED RIGHT KNEE, POSTERIOR VIEW

Anterior cruciate ligament
Femur
Medial condyle
Fibular collateral ligament
Lateral condyle
Tibial collateral ligament
Lateral meniscus
Medial meniscus
Cut tendon of biceps femoris muscle
Posterior cruciate ligament
Head of fibula
Tibia

PLATE 79b EXTENDED RIGHT KNEE, ANTERIOR VIEW

Articular cartilage
Patellar surface
Medial condyle
Lateral condyle
Posterior cruciate ligament
Fibular collateral ligament
Tibial collateral ligament
Lateral meniscus
Medial meniscus
Cut tendon of biceps femoris muscle
Anterior cruciate ligament
Fibula
Tibia

PLATE 80a PROXIMAL END OF RIGHT TIBIA, SUPERIOR VIEW

Articular surface of medial condyle
Tibial tuberosity
Articular surface of lateral condyle
Tubercles of intercondylar eminence

PLATE 80b DISTAL END OF TIBIA AND FIBULA, INFERIOR VIEW

Lateral malleolus (fibula)
Inferior articular surface for ankle joint
Medial malleolus (tibia)

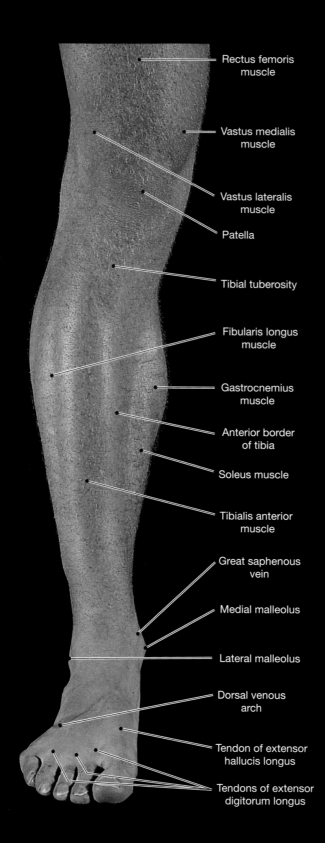

Rectus femoris muscle

Vastus medialis muscle

Vastus lateralis muscle

Patella

Tibial tuberosity

Fibularis longus muscle

Gastrocnemius muscle

Anterior border of tibia

Soleus muscle

Tibialis anterior muscle

Great saphenous vein

Medial malleolus

Lateral malleolus

Dorsal venous arch

Tendon of extensor hallucis longus

Tendons of extensor digitorum longus

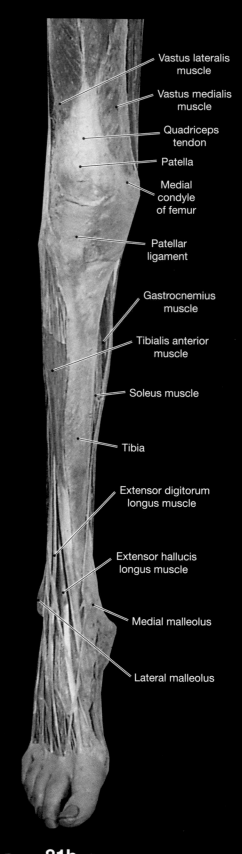

Vastus lateralis muscle

Vastus medialis muscle

Quadriceps tendon

Patella

Medial condyle of femur

Patellar ligament

Gastrocnemius muscle

Tibialis anterior muscle

Soleus muscle

Tibia

Extensor digitorum longus muscle

Extensor hallucis longus muscle

Medial malleolus

Lateral malleolus

PLATE **81a** SURFACE ANATOMY OF THE RIGHT LEG AND FOOT, ANTERIOR VIEW

PLATE **81b** SUPERFICIAL DISSECTION OF THE RIGHT LEG AND FOOT, ANTERIOR VIEW

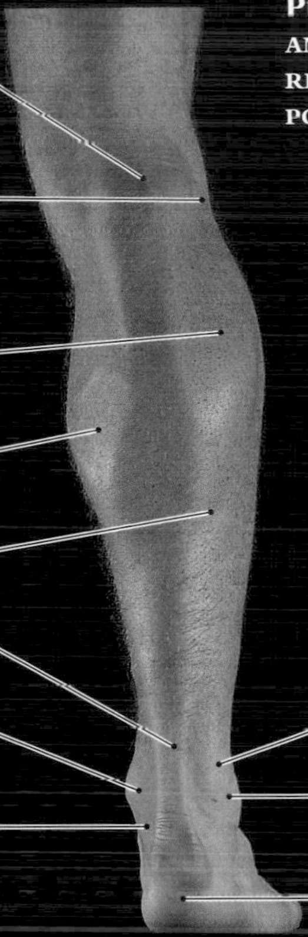

Site for palpation of popliteal artery

Site for palpation of common peroneal nerve

Gastrocnemius muscle, lateral head

Gastrocnemius muscle, medial head

Soleus muscle

Calcaneal tendon

Medial malleolus

Site for palpation of posterior tibial artery

PLATE **82a** SURFACE ANATOMY OF THE RIGHT LEG AND FOOT, POSTERIOR VIEW

Tendon of fibularis longus

Lateral malleolus

Calcaneus

Tendon of gracilis

Tendon of semitendinosus

Tendon of semimembranosus

Gastrocnemius muscle, medial head

Plantaris muscle (cut)

Gastrocnemius muscle, lateral head

Tibial nerve

Tendon of biceps femoris

Common fibular nerve

Plantaris muscle (cut)

Soleus muscle

Tendon of tibialis posterior

Fibularis longus muscle

Calcaneal tendon

Flexor hallucis longus muscle

Flexor digitorum longus muscle

Fibularis brevis muscle

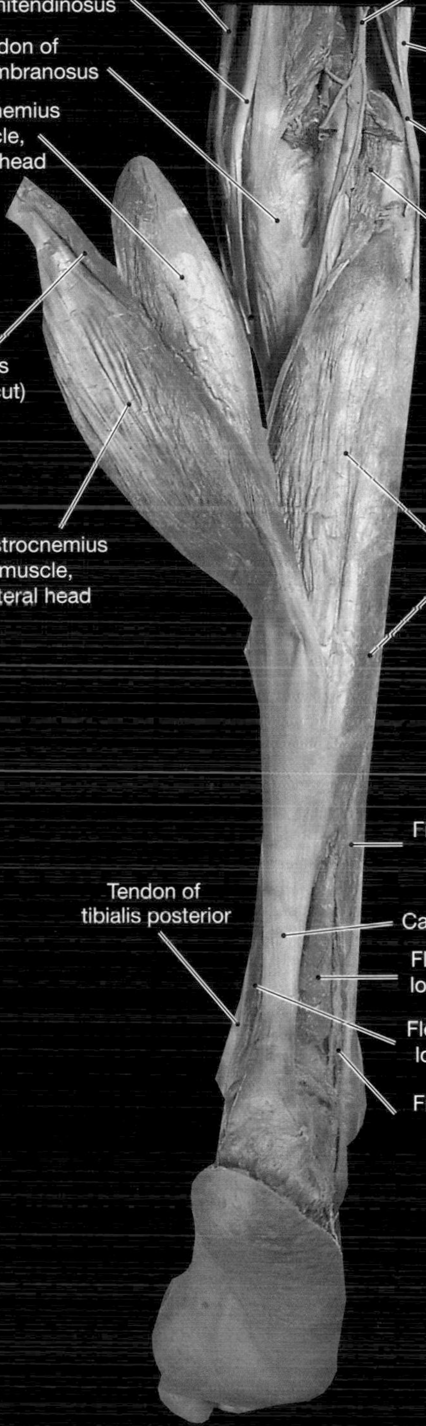

PLATE **82b** SUPERFICIAL DISSECTION OF THE RIGHT LEG AND FOOT, POSTERIOR VIEW

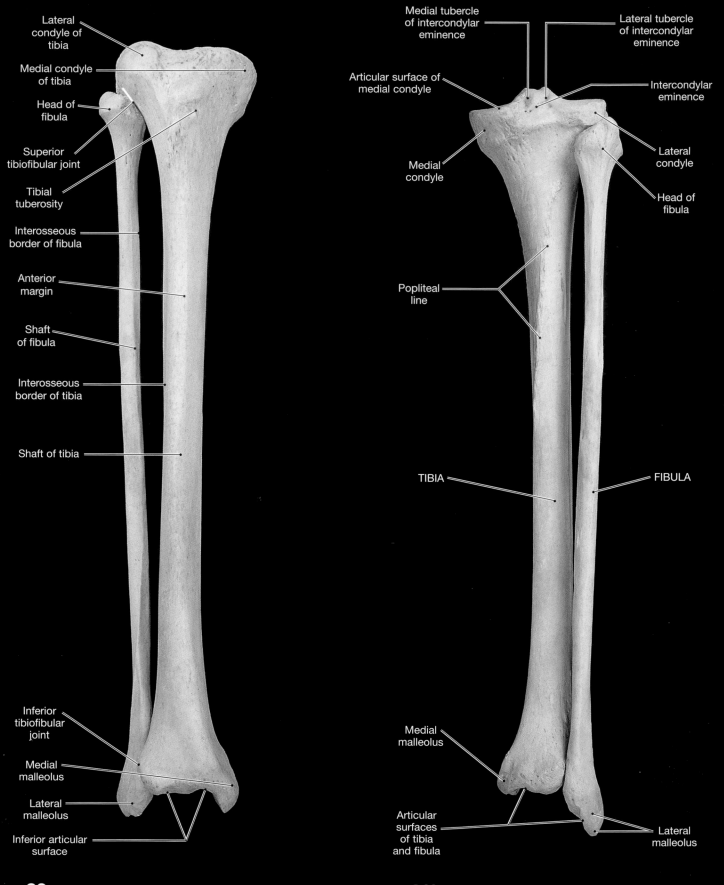

Lateral condyle of tibia

Medial condyle of tibia

Head of fibula

Superior tibiofibular joint

Tibial tuberosity

Interosseous border of fibula

Anterior margin

Shaft of fibula

Interosseous border of tibia

Shaft of tibia

Inferior tibiofibular joint

Medial malleolus

Lateral malleolus

Inferior articular surface

Medial tubercle of intercondylar eminence

Lateral tubercle of intercondylar eminence

Articular surface of medial condyle

Intercondylar eminence

Medial condyle

Lateral condyle

Head of fibula

Popliteal line

TIBIA

FIBULA

Medial malleolus

Articular surfaces of tibia and fibula

Lateral malleolus

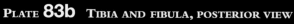

PLATE **83a**   Tibia and fibula, anterior view

PLATE **83b**   Tibia and fibula, posterior view

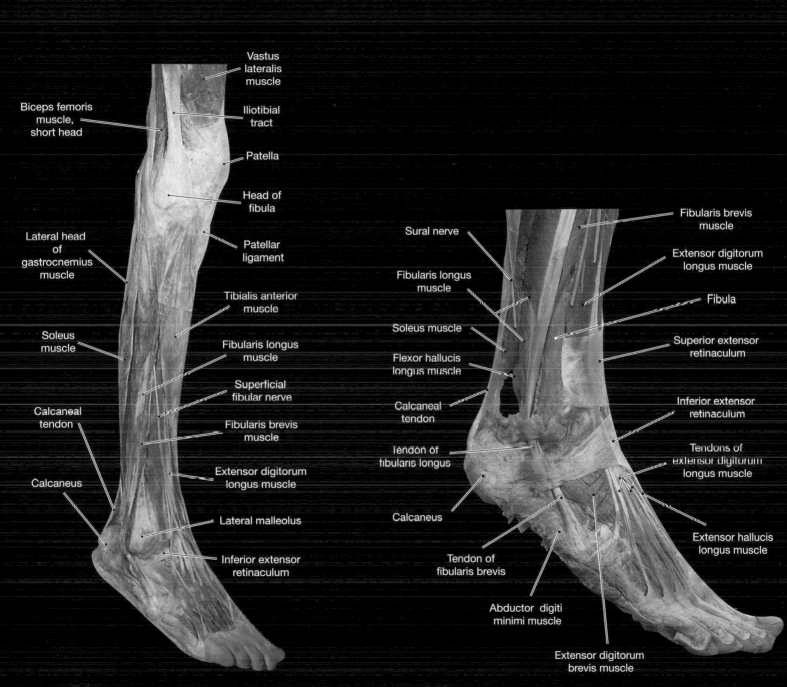

Vastus
lateralis
muscle

Biceps femoris
muscle,
short head

Iliotibial
tract

Patella

Head of
fibula

Lateral head
of
gastrocnemius
muscle

Patellar
ligament

Tibialis anterior
muscle

Soleus
muscle

Fibularis longus
muscle

Superficial
fibular nerve

Calcaneal
tendon

Fibularis brevis
muscle

Calcaneus

Extensor digitorum
longus muscle

Lateral malleolus

Inferior extensor
retinaculum

Sural nerve

Fibularis brevis
muscle

Fibularis longus
muscle

Extensor digitorum
longus muscle

Soleus muscle

Fibula

Flexor hallucis
longus muscle

Superior extensor
retinaculum

Calcaneal
tendon

Inferior extensor
retinaculum

Tendon of
fibularis longus

Tendons of
extensor digitorum
longus muscle

Calcaneus

Tendon of
fibularis brevis

Extensor hallucis
longus muscle

Abductor digiti
minimi muscle

Extensor digitorum
brevis muscle

PLATE 84a SUPERFICIAL DISSECTION OF THE
RIGHT LEG AND FOOT, ANTEROLATERAL VIEW

PLATE 84b SUPERFICIAL DISSECTION OF THE RIGHT FOOT,
LATERAL VIEW

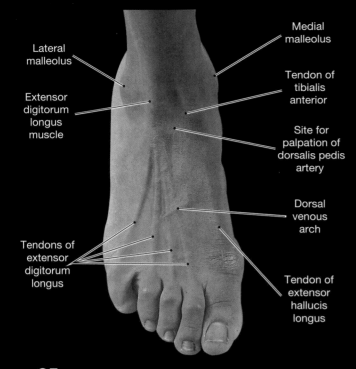

Lateral malleolus

Extensor digitorum longus muscle

Tendons of extensor digitorum longus

Medial malleolus

Tendon of tibialis anterior

Site for palpation of dorsalis pedis artery

Dorsal venous arch

Tendon of extensor hallucis longus

PLATE 85a   SURFACE ANATOMY OF THE RIGHT FOOT, SUPERIOR VIEW

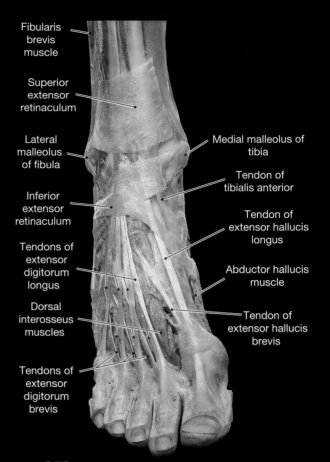

Fibularis brevis muscle

Superior extensor retinaculum

Lateral malleolus of fibula

Inferior extensor retinaculum

Tendons of extensor digitorum longus

Dorsal interosseus muscles

Tendons of extensor digitorum brevis

Medial malleolus of tibia

Tendon of tibialis anterior

Tendon of extensor hallucis longus

Abductor hallucis muscle

Tendon of extensor hallucis brevis

PLATE 85b   SUPERFICIAL DISSECTION OF THE RIGHT FOOT, SUPERIOR VIEW

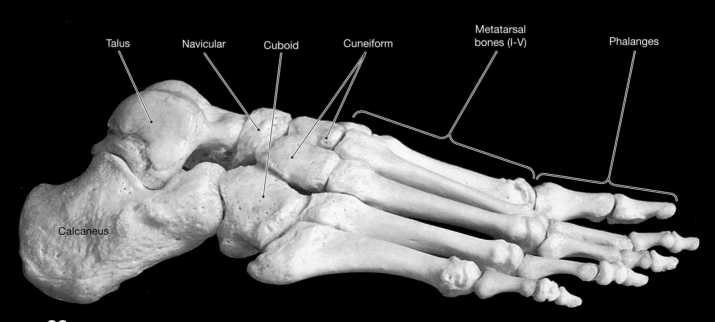

Talus   Navicular   Cuboid   Cuneiform   Metatarsal bones (I-V)   Phalanges

Calcaneus

PLATE 86a   BONES OF THE RIGHT FOOT, LATERAL VIEW

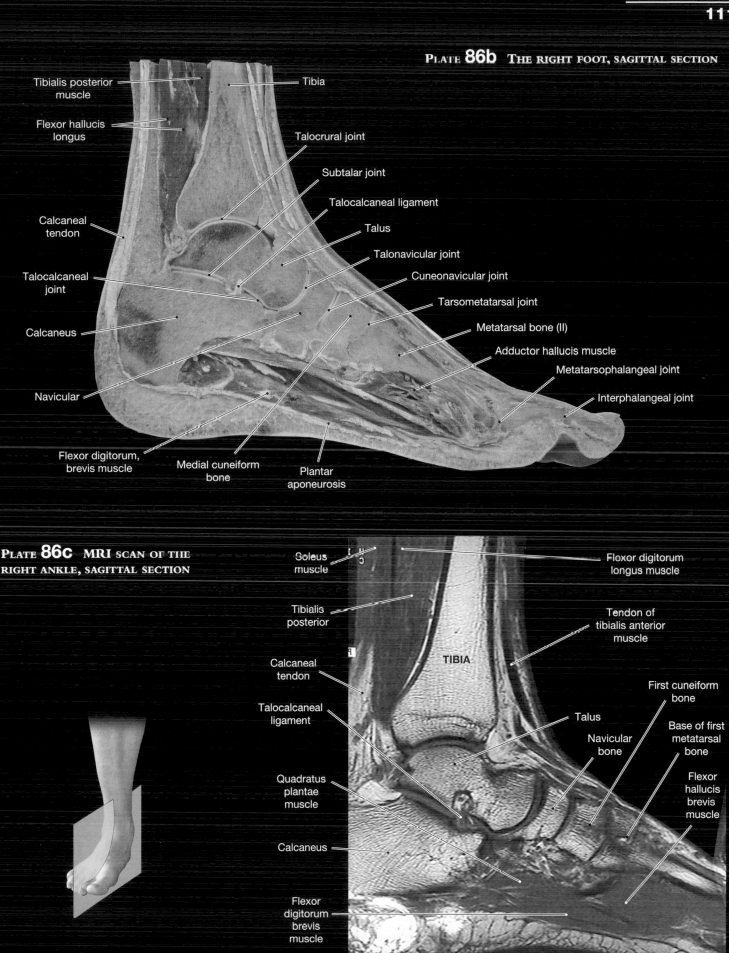

PLATE **86b** THE RIGHT FOOT, SAGITTAL SECTION

Tibialis posterior muscle

Flexor hallucis longus

Calcaneal tendon

Talocalcaneal joint

Calcaneus

Navicular

Flexor digitorum, brevis muscle

Medial cuneiform bone

Plantar aponeurosis

Tibia

Talocrural joint

Subtalar joint

Talocalcaneal ligament

Talus

Talonavicular joint

Cuneonavicular joint

Tarsometatarsal joint

Metatarsal bone (II)

Adductor hallucis muscle

Metatarsophalangeal joint

Interphalangeal joint

PLATE **86c** MRI SCAN OF THE RIGHT ANKLE, SAGITTAL SECTION

Soleus muscle

Tibialis posterior

Calcaneal tendon

Talocalcaneal ligament

Quadratus plantae muscle

Calcaneus

Flexor digitorum brevis muscle

Flexor digitorum longus muscle

Tendon of tibialis anterior muscle

TIBIA

Talus

Navicular bone

First cuneiform bone

Base of first metatarsal bone

Flexor hallucis brevis muscle

PLATE **87a** ANKLE AND FOOT,
POSTERIOR VIEW

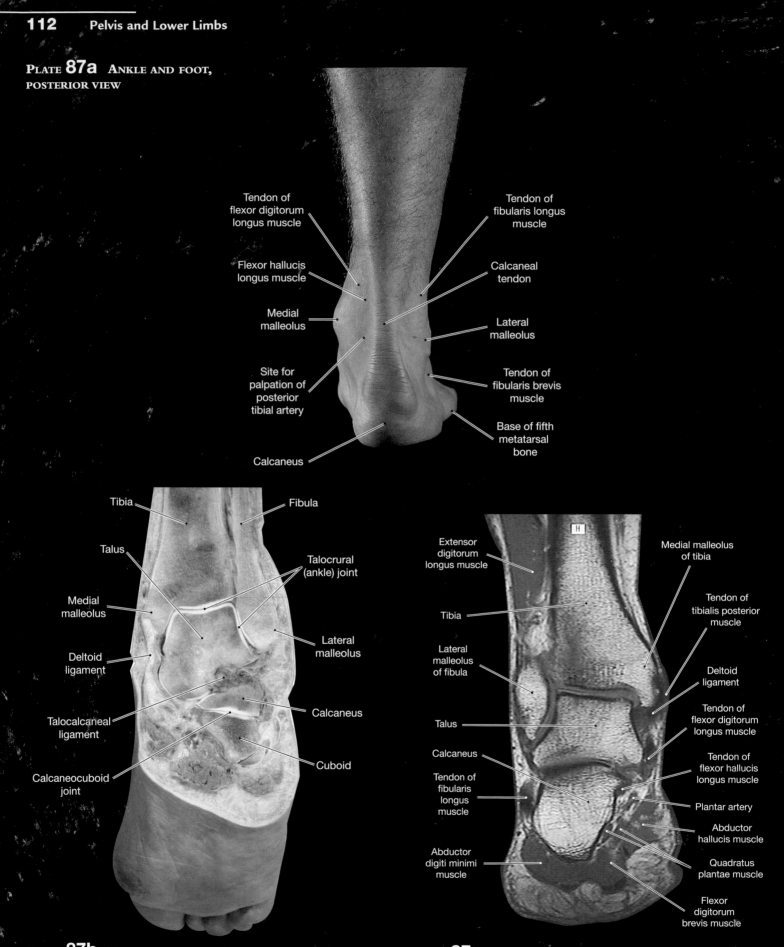

Tendon of
flexor digitorum
longus muscle

Flexor hallucis
longus muscle

Medial
malleolus

Site for
palpation of
posterior
tibial artery

Calcaneus

Tendon of
fibularis longus
muscle

Calcaneal
tendon

Lateral
malleolus

Tendon of
fibularis brevis
muscle

Base of fifth
metatarsal
bone

Tibia

Talus

Medial
malleolus

Deltoid
ligament

Talocalcaneal
ligament

Calcaneocuboid
joint

Fibula

Talocrural
(ankle) joint

Lateral
malleolus

Calcaneus

Cuboid

Extensor
digitorum
longus muscle

Tibia

Lateral
malleolus
of fibula

Talus

Calcaneus

Tendon of
fibularis
longus
muscle

Abductor
digiti minimi
muscle

Medial malleolus
of tibia

Tendon of
tibialis posterior
muscle

Deltoid
ligament

Tendon of
flexor digitorum
longus muscle

Tendon of
flexor hallucis
longus muscle

Plantar artery

Abductor
hallucis muscle

Quadratus
plantae muscle

Flexor
digitorum
brevis muscle

PLATE **87b** FRONTAL SECTION THROUGH THE RIGHT FOOT,
POSTERIOR VIEW

PLATE **87c** MRI SCAN OF THE RIGHT ANKLE, FRONTAL
SECTION

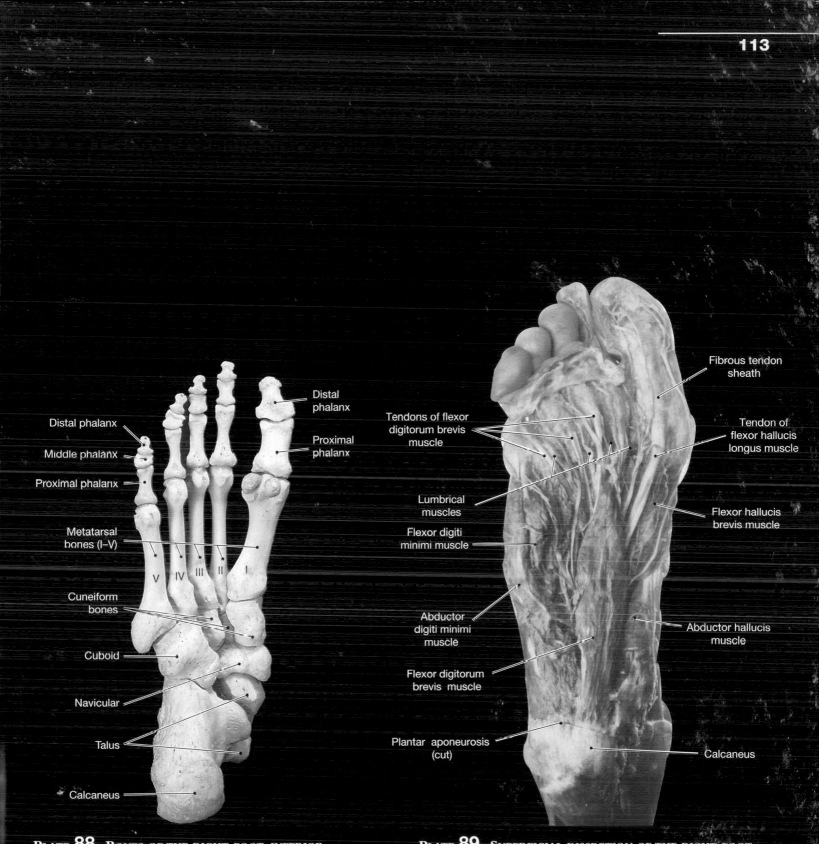

Distal
phalanx

Proximal
phalanx

Distal phalanx

Middle phalanx

Proximal phalanx

Metatarsal
bones (I–V)

V   IV   III   II   I

Cuneiform
bones

Cuboid

Navicular

Talus

Calcaneus

Fibrous tendon
sheath

Tendons of flexor
digitorum brevis
muscle

Tendon of
flexor hallucis
longus muscle

Lumbrical
muscles

Flexor hallucis
brevis muscle

Flexor digiti
minimi muscle

Abductor
digiti minimi
muscle

Abductor hallucis
muscle

Flexor digitorum
brevis muscle

Plantar aponeurosis
(cut)

Calcaneus

**PLATE 88 BONES OF THE RIGHT FOOT, INFERIOR
(PLANTAR) VIEW**

**PLATE 89 SUPERFICIAL DISSECTION OF THE RIGHT FOOT,
PLANTAR VIEW**

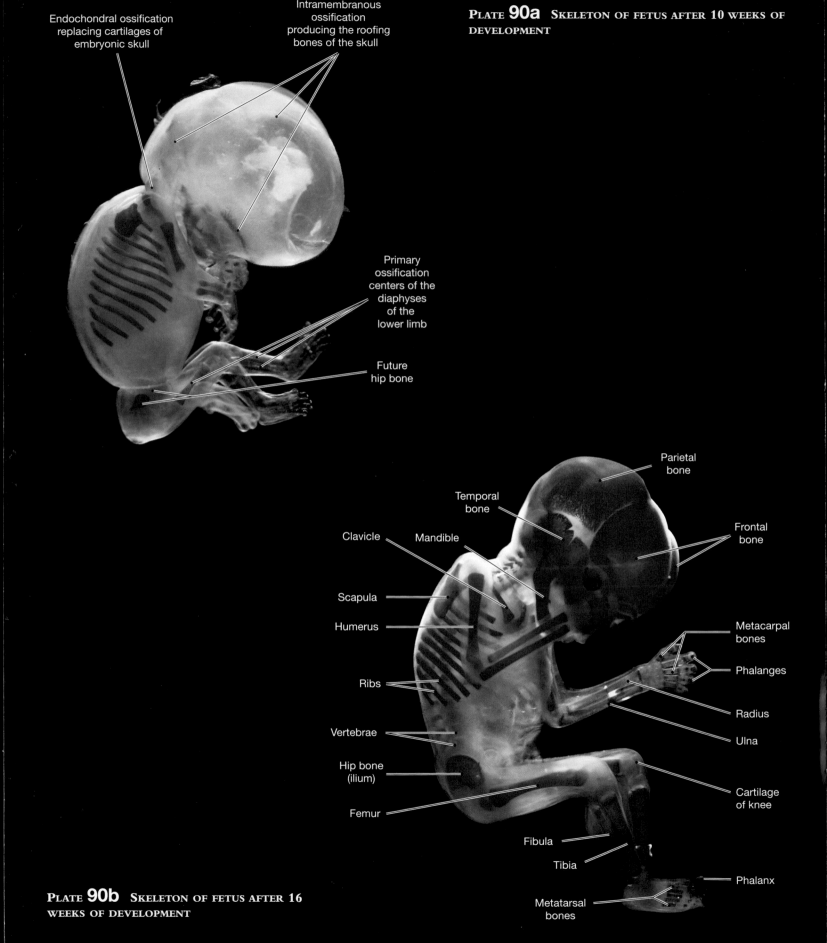

Endochondral ossification replacing cartilages of embryonic skull

Intramembranous ossification producing the roofing bones of the skull

Primary ossification centers of the diaphyses of the lower limb

Future hip bone

Parietal bone

Temporal bone

Clavicle

Mandible

Frontal bone

Scapula

Humerus

Metacarpal bones

Phalanges

Ribs

Radius

Vertebrae

Ulna

Hip bone (ilium)

Femur

Cartilage of knee

Fibula

Tibia

Phalanx

PLATE **90b** SKELETON OF FETUS AFTER **16** WEEKS OF DEVELOPMENT

Metatarsal bones

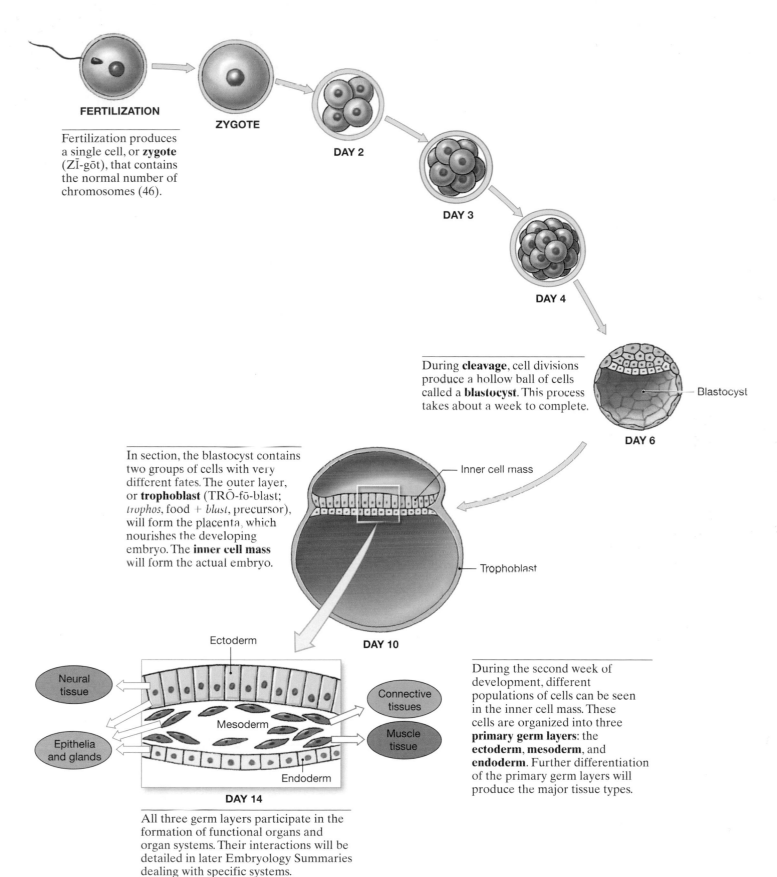

FERTILIZATION

Fertilization produces a single cell, or **zygote** (ZĪ-gōt), that contains the normal number of chromosomes (46).

ZYGOTE

DAY 2

DAY 3

DAY 4

During **cleavage**, cell divisions produce a hollow ball of cells called a **blastocyst**. This process takes about a week to complete.

Blastocyst

DAY 6

In section, the blastocyst contains two groups of cells with very different fates. The outer layer, or **trophoblast** (TRŌ-fō-blast; *trophos*, food + *blast*, precursor), will form the placenta, which nourishes the developing embryo. The **inner cell mass** will form the actual embryo.

Inner cell mass

Trophoblast

DAY 10

Ectoderm

Neural tissue

Epithelia and glands

Mesoderm

Connective tissues

Muscle tissue

Endoderm

DAY 14

During the second week of development, different populations of cells can be seen in the inner cell mass. These cells are organized into three **primary germ layers**: the **ectoderm**, **mesoderm**, and **endoderm**. Further differentiation of the primary germ layers will produce the major tissue types.

All three germ layers participate in the formation of functional organs and organ systems. Their interactions will be detailed in later Embryology Summaries dealing with specific systems.

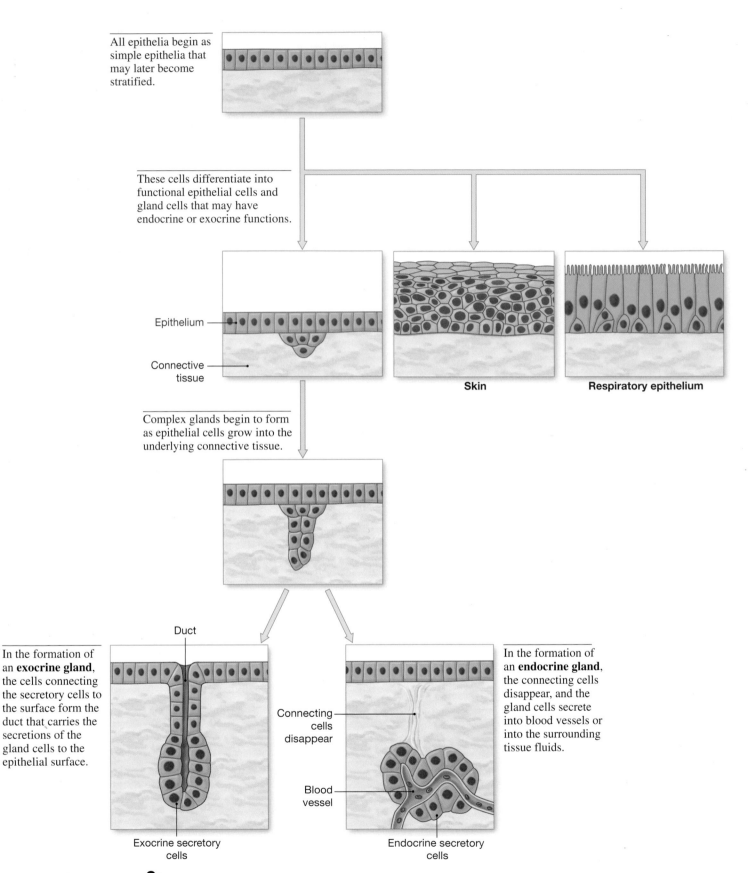

All epithelia begin as simple epithelia that may later become stratified.

These cells differentiate into functional epithelial cells and gland cells that may have endocrine or exocrine functions.

Epithelium

Connective tissue

Skin

Respiratory epithelium

Complex glands begin to form as epithelial cells grow into the underlying connective tissue.

Duct

In the formation of an **exocrine gland**, the cells connecting the secretory cells to the surface form the duct that carries the secretions of the gland cells to the epithelial surface.

Connecting cells disappear

Blood vessel

In the formation of an **endocrine gland**, the connecting cells disappear, and the gland cells secrete into blood vessels or into the surrounding tissue fluids.

Exocrine secretory cells

Endocrine secretory cells

EMBRYOLOGY SUMMARY **2:** THE DEVELOPMENT OF EPITHELIA

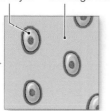

Ectoderm

Mesoderm

Endoderm

Chondrocyte   Cartilage matrix

Chondroblast

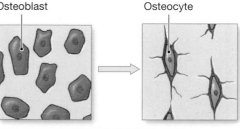

Cartilage develops as mesenchymal cells differentiate into **chondroblasts** that produce cartilage matrix. These cells later become chondrocytes.

Supporting connective tissue

Mesenchyme is the first connective tissue to appear in the developing embryo. Mesenchyme contains star-shaped cells that are separated by a ground substance that contains fine protein filaments. Mesenchyme gives rise to all other forms of connective tissue, and scattered mesenchymal cells in adult connective tissues participate in their repair after injury.

Osteoblast   Osteocyte

Bone formation begins as mesenchymal cells differentiate into **osteoblasts** that lay down the matrix of bone. These cells later become trapped as osteocytes.

Blood   Lymph

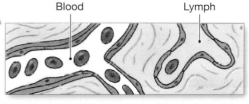

Fluid connective tissues form, as mesenchymal cells create a network of interconnected tubes. Cells trapped in those tubes differentiate into red and white blood cells.

Fluid connective tissue

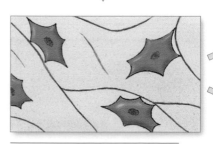

Loose connective tissue

Embryonic connective tissue develops as the density of fibers increases. Embryonic connective tissue may differentiate into any of the connective tissues proper.

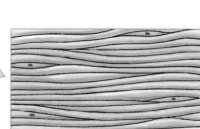

Dense connective tissue

EMBRYOLOGY SUMMARY 3: THE ORIGINS OF CONNECTIVE TISSUES

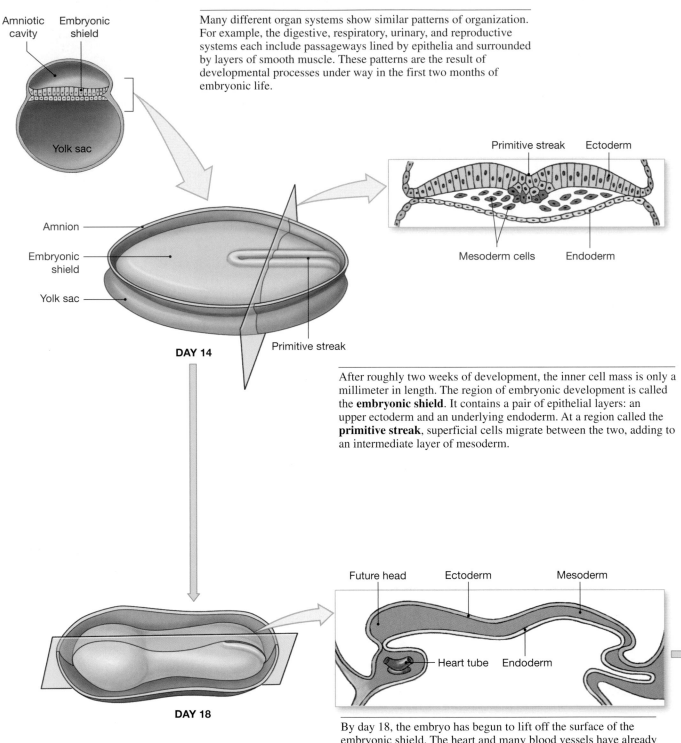

Many different organ systems show similar patterns of organization. For example, the digestive, respiratory, urinary, and reproductive systems each include passageways lined by epithelia and surrounded by layers of smooth muscle. These patterns are the result of developmental processes under way in the first two months of embryonic life.

Amniotic cavity

Embryonic shield

Yolk sac

Primitive streak   Ectoderm

Mesoderm cells   Endoderm

Amnion

Embryonic shield

Yolk sac

DAY 14

Primitive streak

After roughly two weeks of development, the inner cell mass is only a millimeter in length. The region of embryonic development is called the **embryonic shield**. It contains a pair of epithelial layers: an upper ectoderm and an underlying endoderm. At a region called the **primitive streak**, superficial cells migrate between the two, adding to an intermediate layer of mesoderm.

Future head   Ectoderm   Mesoderm

Heart tube   Endoderm

DAY 18

By day 18, the embryo has begun to lift off the surface of the embryonic shield. The heart and many blood vessels have already formed, well ahead of the other organ systems. Unless otherwise noted, discussions of organ system development in subsequent embryology summaries will begin at this stage.

EMBRYOLOGY SUMMARY 4: THE DEVELOPMENT OF ORGAN SYSTEMS

DERIVATIVES OF PRIMARY GERM LAYERS

Ectoderm Forms:
Epidermis and epidermal derivatives of the integumentary system, including hair follicles, nails, and
  glands communicating with the skin surface (sweat, milk, and sebum)
Lining of the mouth, salivary glands, nasal passageways, and anus
Nervous system, including brain and spinal cord
Portions of endocrine system (pituitary gland and parts of adrenal glands)
Portions of skull, pharyngeal arches, and teeth

Mesoderm Forms:
Dermis of integumentary system
Lining of the body cavities (pleural, pericardial, peritoneal)
Muscular, skeletal, cardiovascular, and lymphatic systems
Kidneys and part of the urinary tract
Gonads and most of the reproductive tract
Connective tissues supporting all organ systems
Portions of endocrine system (parts of adrenal glands and endocrine tissues of the reproductive tract)

Endoderm Forms:
Most of the digestive system: epithelium (except mouth and anus), exocrine glands (except
  salivary glands), the liver and pancreas
Most of the respiratory system: epithelium (except nasal passageways) and mucous glands
Portions of urinary and reproductive systems (ducts and the stem cells that produce gametes)
Portions of endocrine system (thymus, thyroid gland, parathyroid glands, and pancreas)

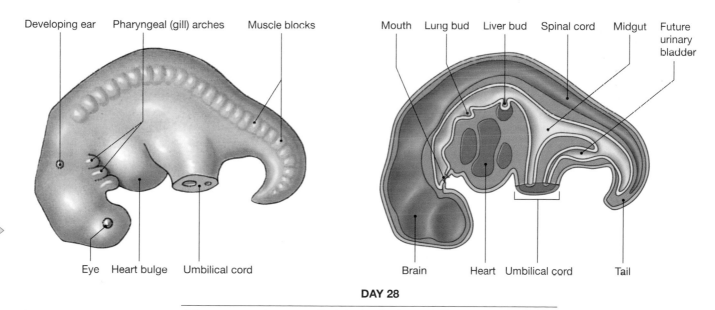

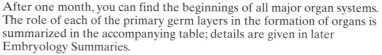

DAY 28

After one month, you can find the beginnings of all major organ systems.
The role of each of the primary germ layers in the formation of organs is
summarized in the accompanying table; details are given in later
Embryology Summaries.

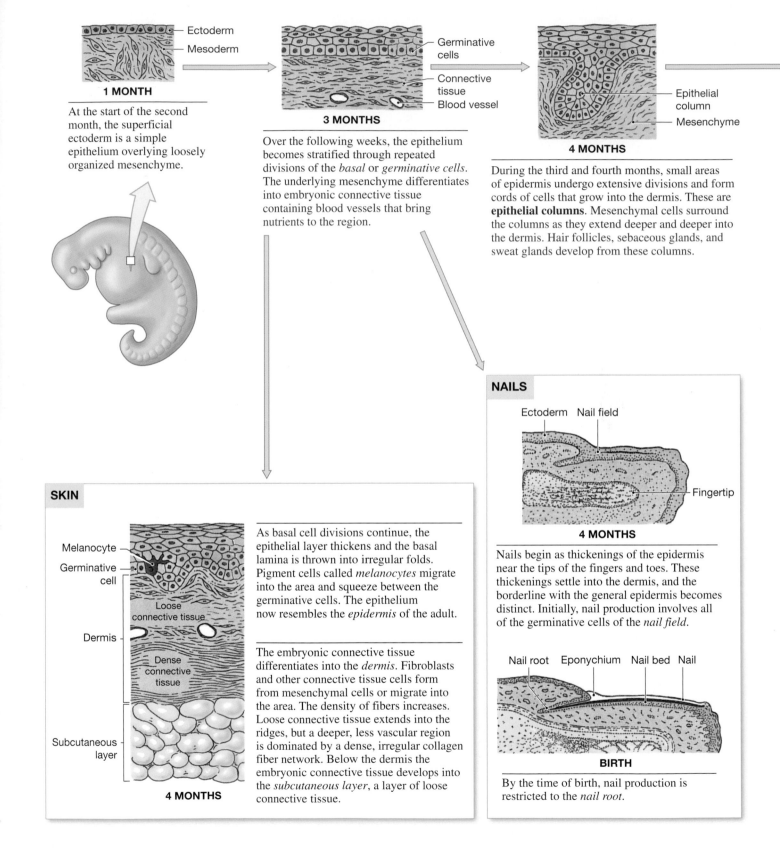

1 MONTH

At the start of the second month, the superficial ectoderm is a simple epithelium overlying loosely organized mesenchyme.

— Ectoderm
— Mesoderm

3 MONTHS

— Germinative cells
— Connective tissue
— Blood vessel

Over the following weeks, the epithelium becomes stratified through repeated divisions of the *basal* or *germinative cells*. The underlying mesenchyme differentiates into embryonic connective tissue containing blood vessels that bring nutrients to the region.

4 MONTHS

— Epithelial column
— Mesenchyme

During the third and fourth months, small areas of epidermis undergo extensive divisions and form cords of cells that grow into the dermis. These are **epithelial columns**. Mesenchymal cells surround the columns as they extend deeper and deeper into the dermis. Hair follicles, sebaceous glands, and sweat glands develop from these columns.

SKIN

Melanocyte
Germinative cell
Loose connective tissue
Dermis
Dense connective tissue
Subcutaneous layer

4 MONTHS

As basal cell divisions continue, the epithelial layer thickens and the basal lamina is thrown into irregular folds. Pigment cells called *melanocytes* migrate into the area and squeeze between the germinative cells. The epithelium now resembles the *epidermis* of the adult.

The embryonic connective tissue differentiates into the *dermis*. Fibroblasts and other connective tissue cells form from mesenchymal cells or migrate into the area. The density of fibers increases. Loose connective tissue extends into the ridges, but a deeper, less vascular region is dominated by a dense, irregular collagen fiber network. Below the dermis the embryonic connective tissue develops into the *subcutaneous layer*, a layer of loose connective tissue.

NAILS

Ectoderm Nail field
Fingertip

4 MONTHS

Nails begin as thickenings of the epidermis near the tips of the fingers and toes. These thickenings settle into the dermis, and the borderline with the general epidermis becomes distinct. Initially, nail production involves all of the germinative cells of the *nail field*.

Nail root Eponychium Nail bed Nail

BIRTH

By the time of birth, nail production is restricted to the *nail root*.

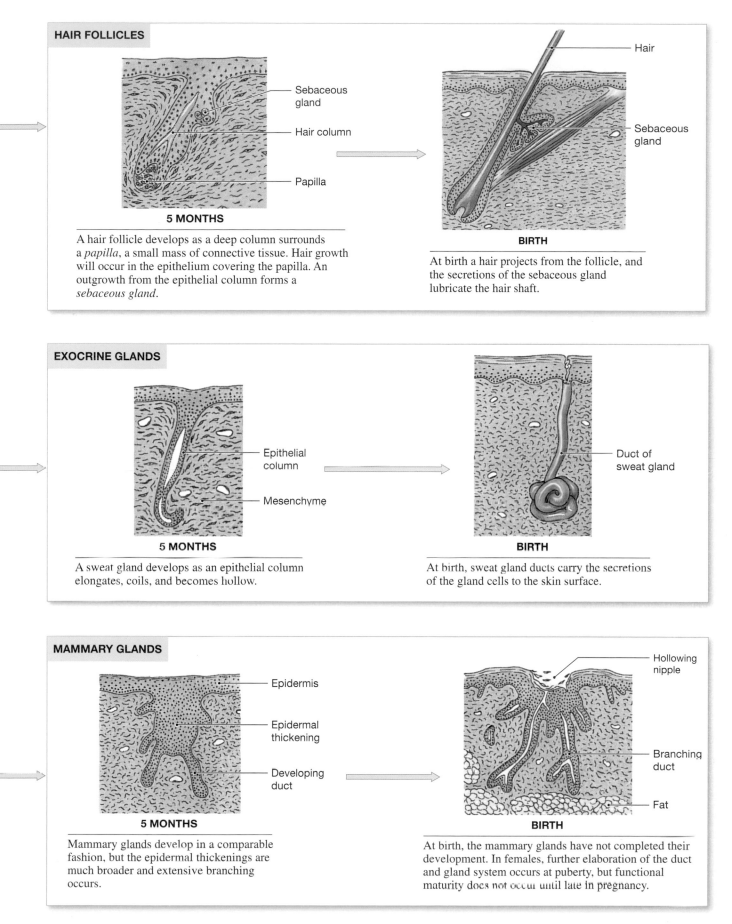

HAIR FOLLICLES

- Sebaceous gland
- Hair column
- Papilla

5 MONTHS

A hair follicle develops as a deep column surrounds a *papilla*, a small mass of connective tissue. Hair growth will occur in the epithelium covering the papilla. An outgrowth from the epithelial column forms a *sebaceous gland*.

- Hair
- Sebaceous gland

BIRTH

At birth a hair projects from the follicle, and the secretions of the sebaceous gland lubricate the hair shaft.

EXOCRINE GLANDS

- Epithelial column
- Mesenchyme

5 MONTHS

A sweat gland develops as an epithelial column elongates, coils, and becomes hollow.

- Duct of sweat gland

BIRTH

At birth, sweat gland ducts carry the secretions of the gland cells to the skin surface.

MAMMARY GLANDS

- Epidermis
- Epidermal thickening
- Developing duct

5 MONTHS

Mammary glands develop in a comparable fashion, but the epidermal thickenings are much broader and extensive branching occurs.

- Hollowing nipple
- Branching duct
- Fat

BIRTH

At birth, the mammary glands have not completed their development. In females, further elaboration of the duct and gland system occurs at puberty, but functional maturity does not occur until late in pregnancy.

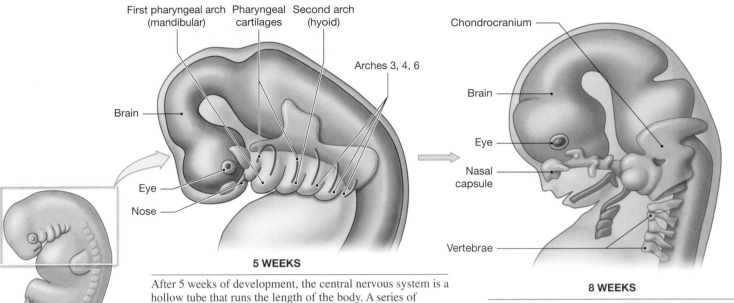

5-WEEK EMBRYO

5 WEEKS

After 5 weeks of development, the central nervous system is a hollow tube that runs the length of the body. A series of cartilages appears in the mesenchyme of the head beneath and alongside the expanding brain and around the developing nose, eyes, and ears. These cartilages are shown in light blue. Five additional pairs of cartilages develop in the walls of the pharynx. These cartilages, shown in dark blue, are located within the **pharyngeal**, or **branchial, arches**. (*Branchial* refers to gills—in fish the caudal arches develop into skeletal supports for the gills.) The first arch, or **mandibular arch**, is the largest.

8 WEEKS

The cartilages associated with the brain enlarge and fuse, forming a cartilaginous **chondrocranium** (kon-drō-KRĀ-nē-um; *chondros*, cartilage + *cranium*, skull) that cradles the brain and sense organs. At 8 weeks its walls and floor are incomplete, and there is no roof.

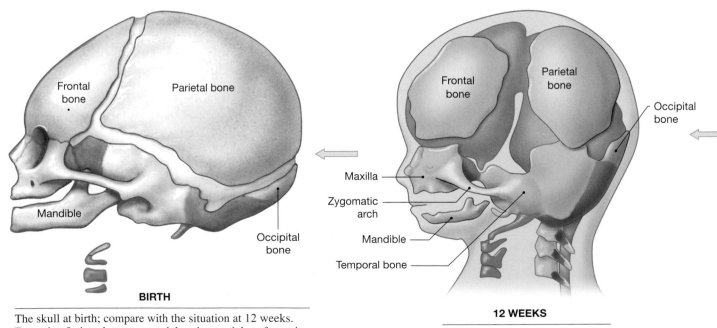

BIRTH

The skull at birth; compare with the situation at 12 weeks. Extensive fusions have occurred, but the cranial roof remains incomplete. (For further details, *see Figure 7–15, p. 230 of the text.*)

12 WEEKS

After 12 weeks ossification is well under way in the cranium and face. Compare with Plate 90b, page 114.

EMBRYOLOGY SUMMARY 6: THE DEVELOPMENT OF THE SKULL

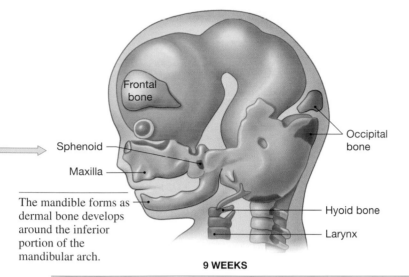

Sphenoid

Maxilla

The mandible forms as dermal bone develops around the inferior portion of the mandibular arch.

Frontal bone

Occipital bone

Hyoid bone

Larynx

9 WEEKS

During the ninth week, numerous centers of endochondral ossification appear within the chondrocranium. These centers are shown in red. Gradually, the frontal and parietal bones of the cranial roof appear as intramembranous ossification begins in the overlying dermis. As these centers (beige) enlarge and expand, extensive fusions occur.

The dorsal portion of the mandibular arch fuses with the chondrocranium. The fused cartilages do not ossify; instead, osteoblasts begin sheathing them in dermal bone. On each side this sheath fuses with a bone developing at the entrance to the nasal cavity, producing the two maxillae. Ossification centers in the roof of the mouth spread to form the palatine processes and later fuse with the maxillae.

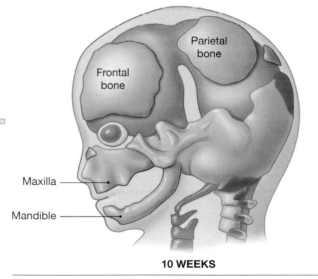

Parietal bone

Frontal bone

Maxilla

Mandible

10 WEEKS

The second arch, or **hyoid arch**, forms near the temporal bones. Fusion of the superior tips of the hyoid with the temporals forms the styloid processes. The ventral portion of the hyoid arch ossifies as the hyoid bone. The third arch fuses with the hyoid, and the fourth and sixth arches form laryngeal cartilages.

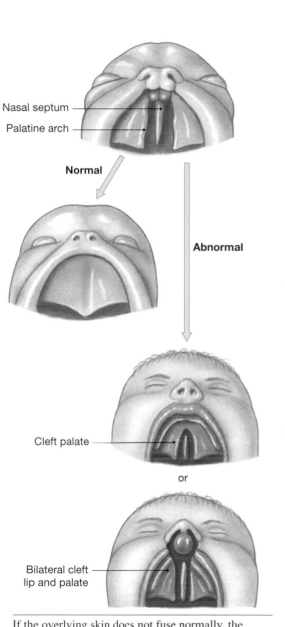

Nasal septum

Palatine arch

Normal

Abnormal

Cleft palate

or

Bilateral cleft lip and palate

If the overlying skin does not fuse normally, the result is a **cleft lip**. Cleft lips affect roughly one birth in a thousand. A split extending into the orbit and palate is called a **cleft palate**. Cleft palates are half as common as cleft lips. Both conditions can be corrected surgically.

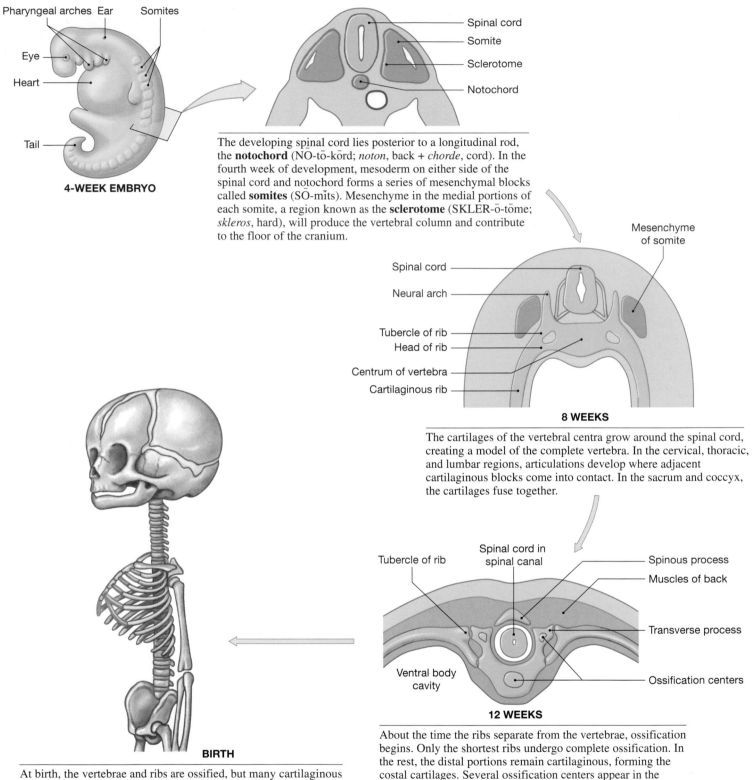

4-WEEK EMBRYO

Pharyngeal arches   Ear   Somites

Eye

Heart

Tail

Spinal cord
Somite
Sclerotome
Notochord

The developing spinal cord lies posterior to a longitudinal rod, the **notochord** (NŌ-tō-kōrd; *noton*, back + *chorde*, cord). In the fourth week of development, mesoderm on either side of the spinal cord and notochord forms a series of mesenchymal blocks called **somites** (SŌ-mīts). Mesenchyme in the medial portions of each somite, a region known as the **sclerotome** (SKLER-ō-tōme; *skleros*, hard), will produce the vertebral column and contribute to the floor of the cranium.

Mesenchyme of somite

Spinal cord
Neural arch

Tubercle of rib
Head of rib
Centrum of vertebra
Cartilaginous rib

8 WEEKS

The cartilages of the vertebral centra grow around the spinal cord, creating a model of the complete vertebra. In the cervical, thoracic, and lumbar regions, articulations develop where adjacent cartilaginous blocks come into contact. In the sacrum and coccyx, the cartilages fuse together.

Tubercle of rib

Spinal cord in spinal canal

Spinous process
Muscles of back

Transverse process

Ventral body cavity

Ossification centers

12 WEEKS

About the time the ribs separate from the vertebrae, ossification begins. Only the shortest ribs undergo complete ossification. In the rest, the distal portions remain cartilaginous, forming the costal cartilages. Several ossification centers appear in the sternum, but fusion gradually reduces the number.

BIRTH

At birth, the vertebrae and ribs are ossified, but many cartilaginous areas remain. For example, the anterior portions of the ribs remain cartilaginous. Additional growth will occur for many years; in vertebrae, the bases of the neural arches enlarge until ages 3–6, and the spinal processes and vertebral bodies grow until ages 18–25.

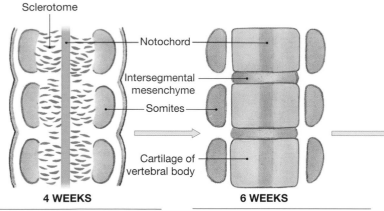

Sclerotome

Notochord

Intersegmental mesenchyme

Somites

Cartilage of vertebral body

4 WEEKS

Cells of the sclerotomal segments migrate away from the somites and cluster around the notochord.

6 WEEKS

The migrating cells differentiate into chondroblasts and produce a series of cartilaginous blocks that surround the notochord. These cartilages, which will develop into the vertebral centra, are separated by patches of mesenchyme.

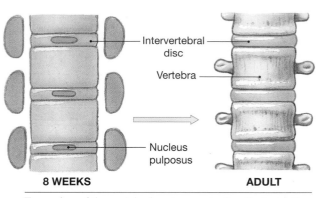

Intervertebral disc

Vertebra

Nucleus pulposus

8 WEEKS

ADULT

Expansion of the vertebral centra eventually eliminates the notochord, but it remains intact between adjacent vertebrae, forming the *nucleus pulposus* of the intervertebral discs. Later, surrounding mesenchymal cells differentiate into chondroblasts and produce the fibrous cartilage of the *anulus fibrosus*.

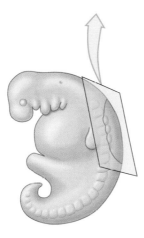

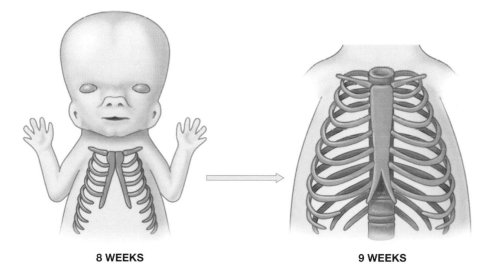

8 WEEKS

9 WEEKS

Rib cartilages expand away from the developing transverse processes of the vertebrae. At first they are continuous, but by week 8 the ribs have separated from the vertebrae. Ribs form at every vertebra, but in the cervical, lumbar, sacral, and coccygeal regions they remain small and later fuse with the growing vertebrae. The ribs of the thoracic vertebrae continue to enlarge, following the curvature of the body wall. When they reach the ventral midline, they fuse with the cartilages of the sternum.

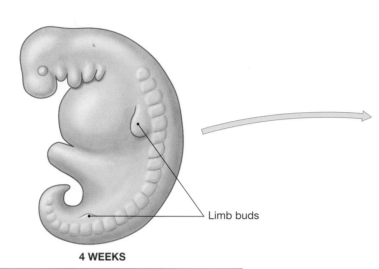

4 WEEKS

In the fourth week of development, ridges appear along the flanks of the embryo, extending from just behind the throat to just before the anus. These ridges form as mesodermal cells congregate beneath the ectoderm of the flank. Mesoderm gradually accumulates at the end of each ridge, forming two pairs of limb buds.

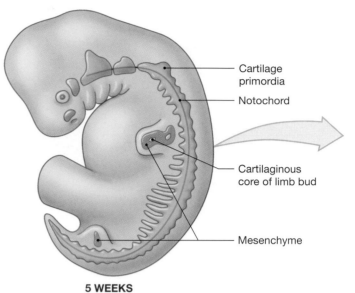

5 WEEKS

After 5 weeks of development, the pectoral limb buds have a cartilaginous core and scapular cartilages are developing in the mesenchyme of the trunk.

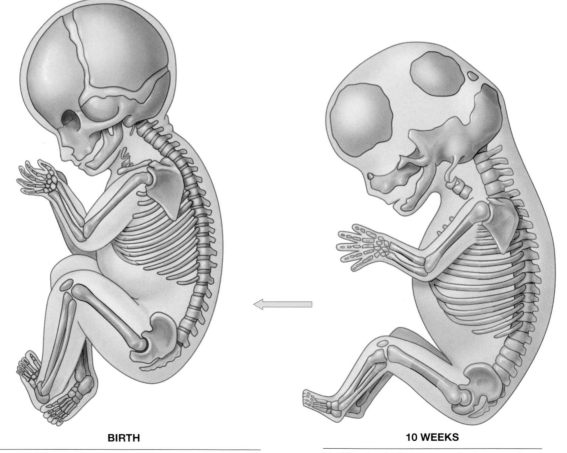

BIRTH

The skeleton of a newborn infant. Note the extensive areas of cartilage (blue) in the humeral head, in the wrist, between the bones of the palm and fingers, and in the hips. Notice the appearance of the axial skeleton, with reference to the two previous Embryology Summaries.

10 WEEKS

Ossification in the embryonic skeleton after approximately 10 weeks of development. The shafts of the limb bones are undergoing rapid ossification, but the distal bones of the carpus and tarsus remain cartilaginous.

EMBRYOLOGY SUMMARY 8: THE DEVELOPMENT OF THE APPENDICULAR SKELETON

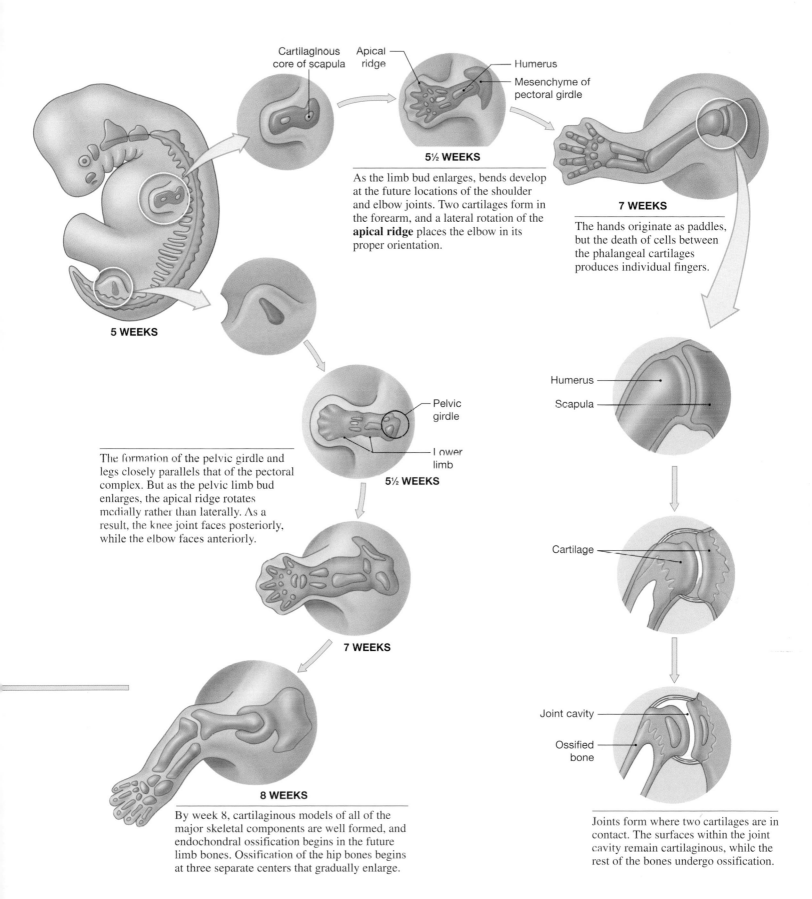

Cartilaginous core of scapula

Apical ridge

Humerus

Mesenchyme of pectoral girdle

5½ WEEKS

As the limb bud enlarges, bends develop at the future locations of the shoulder and elbow joints. Two cartilages form in the forearm, and a lateral rotation of the **apical ridge** places the elbow in its proper orientation.

7 WEEKS

The hands originate as paddles, but the death of cells between the phalangeal cartilages produces individual fingers.

5 WEEKS

Pelvic girdle

Lower limb

5½ WEEKS

The formation of the pelvic girdle and legs closely parallels that of the pectoral complex. But as the pelvic limb bud enlarges, the apical ridge rotates medially rather than laterally. As a result, the knee joint faces posteriorly, while the elbow faces anteriorly.

7 WEEKS

8 WEEKS

By week 8, cartilaginous models of all of the major skeletal components are well formed, and endochondral ossification begins in the future limb bones. Ossification of the hip bones begins at three separate centers that gradually enlarge.

Humerus

Scapula

Cartilage

Joint cavity

Ossified bone

Joints form where two cartilages are in contact. The surfaces within the joint cavity remain cartilaginous, while the rest of the bones undergo ossification.

Near the head, mesoderm forms skeletal muscle associated with the pharyngeal arches.

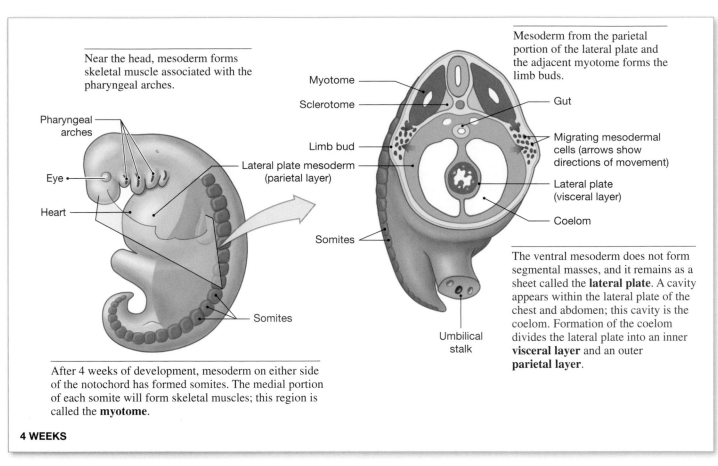

Pharyngeal arches

Eye

Heart

Lateral plate mesoderm (parietal layer)

Somites

Myotome

Sclerotome

Limb bud

Somites

Mesoderm from the parietal portion of the lateral plate and the adjacent myotome forms the limb buds.

Gut

Migrating mesodermal cells (arrows show directions of movement)

Lateral plate (visceral layer)

Coelom

Umbilical stalk

The ventral mesoderm does not form segmental masses, and it remains as a sheet called the **lateral plate**. A cavity appears within the lateral plate of the chest and abdomen; this cavity is the coelom. Formation of the coelom divides the lateral plate into an inner **visceral layer** and an outer **parietal layer**.

After 4 weeks of development, mesoderm on either side of the notochord has formed somites. The medial portion of each somite will form skeletal muscles; this region is called the **myotome**.

4 WEEKS

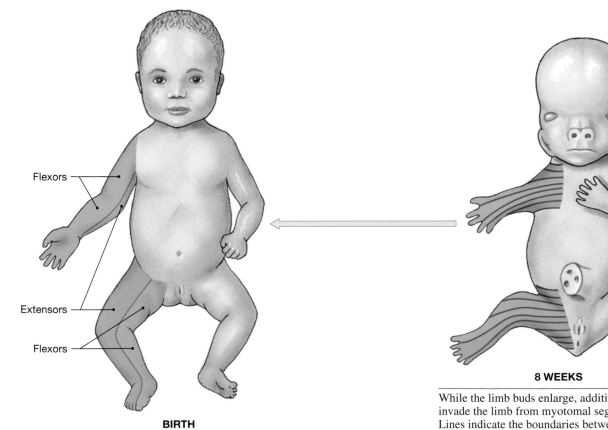

Flexors

Extensors

Flexors

BIRTH

Rotation of the arm and leg buds produces a change in the position of these masses relative to the body axis.

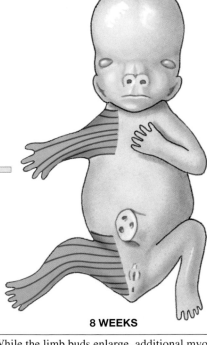

8 WEEKS

While the limb buds enlarge, additional myoblasts invade the limb from myotomal segments nearby. Lines indicate the boundaries between myotomes providing myoblasts to the limb.

EMBRYOLOGY SUMMARY 9: THE DEVELOPMENT OF THE MUSCULAR SYSTEM

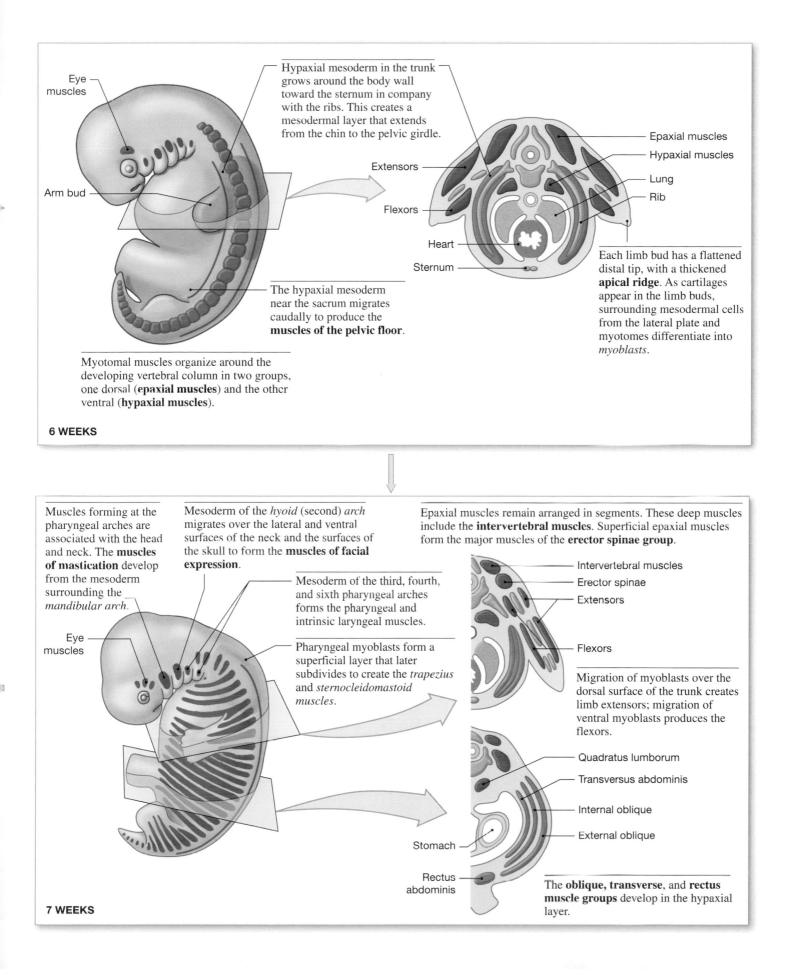

Eye muscles

Hypaxial mesoderm in the trunk grows around the body wall toward the sternum in company with the ribs. This creates a mesodermal layer that extends from the chin to the pelvic girdle.

Epaxial muscles

Hypaxial muscles

Extensors

Lung

Arm bud

Rib

Flexors

Heart

Sternum

Each limb bud has a flattened distal tip, with a thickened **apical ridge**. As cartilages appear in the limb buds, surrounding mesodermal cells from the lateral plate and myotomes differentiate into *myoblasts*.

The hypaxial mesoderm near the sacrum migrates caudally to produce the **muscles of the pelvic floor**.

Myotomal muscles organize around the developing vertebral column in two groups, one dorsal (**epaxial muscles**) and the other ventral (**hypaxial muscles**).

6 WEEKS

Muscles forming at the pharyngeal arches are associated with the head and neck. The **muscles of mastication** develop from the mesoderm surrounding the *mandibular arch*.

Mesoderm of the *hyoid* (second) *arch* migrates over the lateral and ventral surfaces of the neck and the surfaces of the skull to form the **muscles of facial expression**.

Epaxial muscles remain arranged in segments. These deep muscles include the **intervertebral muscles**. Superficial epaxial muscles form the major muscles of the **erector spinae group**.

Mesoderm of the third, fourth, and sixth pharyngeal arches forms the pharyngeal and intrinsic laryngeal muscles.

Intervertebral muscles

Erector spinae

Extensors

Eye muscles

Flexors

Pharyngeal myoblasts form a superficial layer that later subdivides to create the *trapezius* and *sternocleidomastoid muscles*.

Migration of myoblasts over the dorsal surface of the trunk creates limb extensors; migration of ventral myoblasts produces the flexors.

Quadratus lumborum

Transversus abdominis

Internal oblique

External oblique

Stomach

Rectus abdominis

The **oblique, transverse,** and **rectus muscle groups** develop in the hypaxial layer.

7 WEEKS

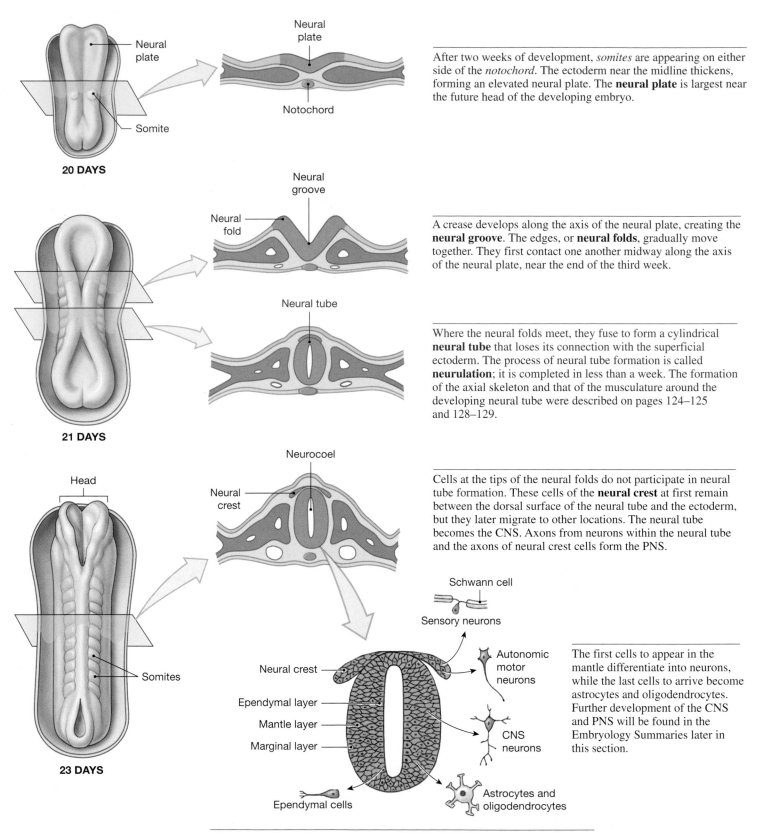

20 DAYS

After two weeks of development, *somites* are appearing on either side of the *notochord*. The ectoderm near the midline thickens, forming an elevated neural plate. The **neural plate** is largest near the future head of the developing embryo.

21 DAYS

A crease develops along the axis of the neural plate, creating the **neural groove**. The edges, or **neural folds**, gradually move together. They first contact one another midway along the axis of the neural plate, near the end of the third week.

Where the neural folds meet, they fuse to form a cylindrical **neural tube** that loses its connection with the superficial ectoderm. The process of neural tube formation is called **neurulation**; it is completed in less than a week. The formation of the axial skeleton and that of the musculature around the developing neural tube were described on pages 124–125 and 128–129.

Cells at the tips of the neural folds do not participate in neural tube formation. These cells of the **neural crest** at first remain between the dorsal surface of the neural tube and the ectoderm, but they later migrate to other locations. The neural tube becomes the CNS. Axons from neurons within the neural tube and the axons of neural crest cells form the PNS.

23 DAYS

The first cells to appear in the mantle differentiate into neurons, while the last cells to arrive become astrocytes and oligodendrocytes. Further development of the CNS and PNS will be found in the Embryology Summaries later in this section.

The neural tube increases in thickness as its epithelial lining undergoes repeated mitoses. By the middle of the fifth developmental week, there are three distinct layers. The **ependymal layer** lines the enclosed cavity, or **neurocoel**. The ependymal cells continue their mitotic activities, and daughter cells create the surrounding **mantle layer**. Axons from developing neurons form a superficial **marginal layer**.

EMBRYOLOGY SUMMARY **10:** AN INTRODUCTION TO THE DEVELOPMENT OF THE NERVOUS SYSTEM

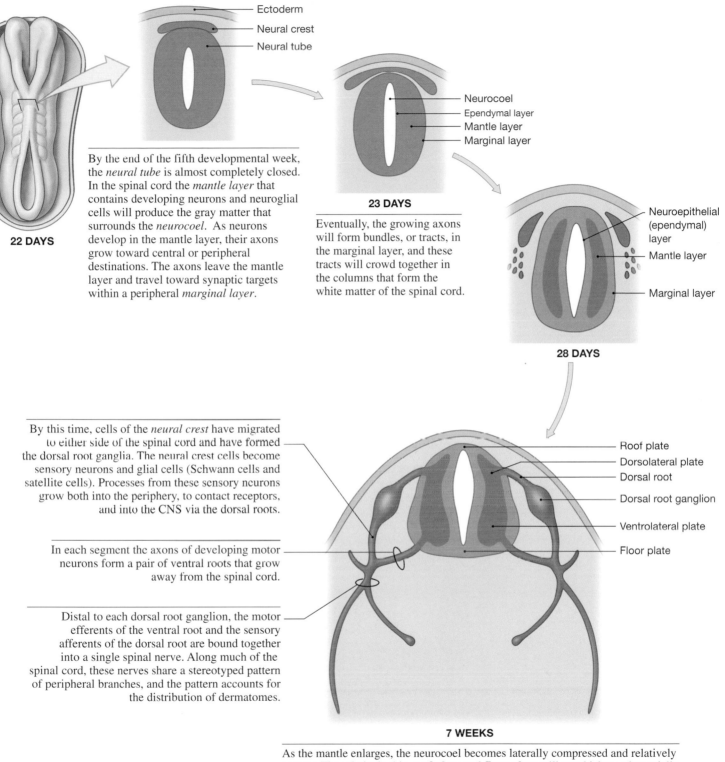

Ectoderm
Neural crest
Neural tube

22 DAYS

By the end of the fifth developmental week, the *neural tube* is almost completely closed. In the spinal cord the *mantle layer* that contains developing neurons and neuroglial cells will produce the gray matter that surrounds the *neurocoel*. As neurons develop in the mantle layer, their axons grow toward central or peripheral destinations. The axons leave the mantle layer and travel toward synaptic targets within a peripheral *marginal layer*.

23 DAYS

Neurocoel
Ependymal layer
Mantle layer
Marginal layer

Eventually, the growing axons will form bundles, or tracts, in the marginal layer, and these tracts will crowd together in the columns that form the white matter of the spinal cord.

28 DAYS

Neuroepithelial (ependymal) layer
Mantle layer
Marginal layer

By this time, cells of the *neural crest* have migrated to either side of the spinal cord and have formed the dorsal root ganglia. The neural crest cells become sensory neurons and glial cells (Schwann cells and satellite cells). Processes from these sensory neurons grow both into the periphery, to contact receptors, and into the CNS via the dorsal roots.

In each segment the axons of developing motor neurons form a pair of ventral roots that grow away from the spinal cord.

Distal to each dorsal root ganglion, the motor efferents of the ventral root and the sensory afferents of the dorsal root are bound together into a single spinal nerve. Along much of the spinal cord, these nerves share a stereotyped pattern of peripheral branches, and the pattern accounts for the distribution of dermatomes.

Roof plate
Dorsolateral plate
Dorsal root
Dorsal root ganglion
Ventrolateral plate
Floor plate

7 WEEKS

As the mantle enlarges, the neurocoel becomes laterally compressed and relatively narrow. The relatively thin **roof plate** and **floor plate** will not thicken substantially, but the **dorsolateral** and **ventrolateral plates** enlarge rapidly. Neurons developing within the dorsolateral plate will receive and relay sensory information, while those in the ventrolateral region will develop into motor neurons.

EMBRYOLOGY SUMMARY 11: THE DEVELOPMENT OF THE SPINAL CORD AND SPINAL NERVES—PART I

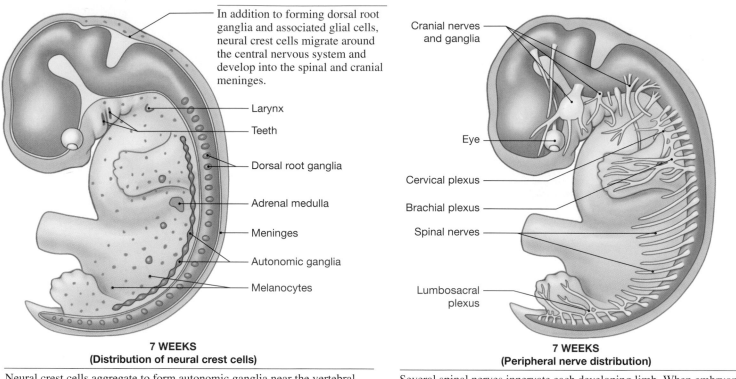

In addition to forming dorsal root ganglia and associated glial cells, neural crest cells migrate around the central nervous system and develop into the spinal and cranial meninges.

- Larynx
- Teeth
- Dorsal root ganglia
- Adrenal medulla
- Meninges
- Autonomic ganglia
- Melanocytes

Cranial nerves and ganglia

- Eye
- Cervical plexus
- Brachial plexus
- Spinal nerves
- Lumbosacral plexus

7 WEEKS
(Distribution of neural crest cells)

7 WEEKS
(Peripheral nerve distribution)

Neural crest cells aggregate to form autonomic ganglia near the vertebral column and in peripheral organs. Migrating neural crest cells contribute to the formation of teeth and form the laryngeal cartilages, melanocytes of the skin, the skull, connective tissues around the eye, the intrinsic muscles of the eye, Schwann cells, satellite cells, and the adrenal medullae.

Several spinal nerves innervate each developing limb. When embryonic muscle cells migrate away from the myotome, the nerves grow right along with them. If a large muscle in the adult is derived from several myotomal blocks, connective tissue partitions will often mark the original boundaries, and the innervation will always involve more than one spinal nerve.

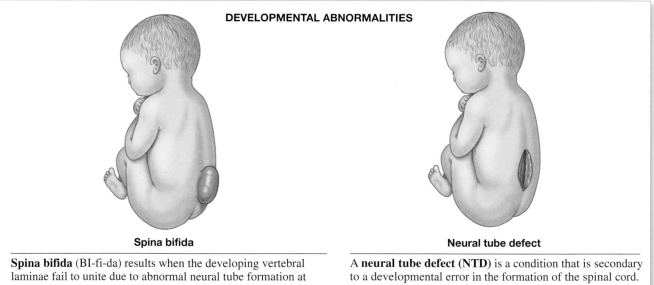

DEVELOPMENTAL ABNORMALITIES

Spina bifida

Neural tube defect

Spina bifida (BI-fi-da) results when the developing vertebral laminae fail to unite due to abnormal neural tube formation at that site. The neural arch is incomplete, and the meninges bulge outward beneath the skin of the back. The extent of the abnormality determines the severity of the defects. In mild cases, the condition may pass unnoticed; extreme cases involve much of the length of the vertebral column.

A **neural tube defect (NTD)** is a condition that is secondary to a developmental error in the formation of the spinal cord. Instead of forming a hollow tube, a portion of the spinal cord develops as a broad plate. This is often associated with spina bifida. Neural tube defects affect roughly one individual in 1000; prenatal testing can detect the existence of these defects with an 80–85 percent success rate.

Before proceeding, briefly review the summaries of skull formation, vertebral column development, and development of the spinal cord in the previous Embryology Summaries.

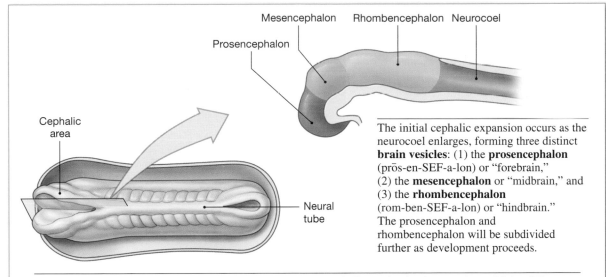

Mesencephalon   Rhombencephalon   Neurocoel

Prosencephalon

The initial cephalic expansion occurs as the neurocoel enlarges, forming three distinct **brain vesicles**: (1) the **prosencephalon** (prōs-en-SEF-a-lon) or "forebrain," (2) the **mesencephalon** or "midbrain," and (3) the **rhombencephalon** (rom-ben-SEF-a-lon) or "hindbrain." The prosencephalon and rhombencephalon will be subdivided further as development proceeds.

Cephalic area

Neural tube

Even before **neural tube** formation has been completed, the cephalic portion begins to enlarge. Major differences in brain versus spinal cord development include (1) early breakdown of mantle (gray matter) and marginal (white matter) organization; (2) appearance of areas of neural cortex; (3) differential growth between and within specific regions; (4) appearance of characteristic bends and folds; and (5) loss of obvious segmental organization.

23 DAYS

Mesencephalon   Metencephalon

Myelencephalon

Diencephalon

Telencephalon

The rhombencephalon first subdivides into the **metencephalon** (met-en-SEF-a-lon; *meta*, after) and the **myelencephalon** (mi-el-ēn-SEF-a-lon; *myelon*, spinal cord).

The prosencephalon forms the **telecephalon** (tel-en-SEF-a-lon; *telos*, end + *enkephalos*, brain) and the **diencephalon**. The telencephalon begins as a pair of swellings near the rostral, dorsolateral border of the prosencephalon.

4 WEEKS

Cranial nerves develop as sensory ganglia and link peripheral receptors with the brain, and motor fibers grow out of developing cranial nuclei. Special sensory neurons of cranial nerves N I, II, and VIII develop in association with the developing receptors. The somatic motor nerves (N III, IV, and VI) grow to the eye muscles; the mixed nerves (N V, VII, IX, and X) innervate the **pharyngeal arches**.

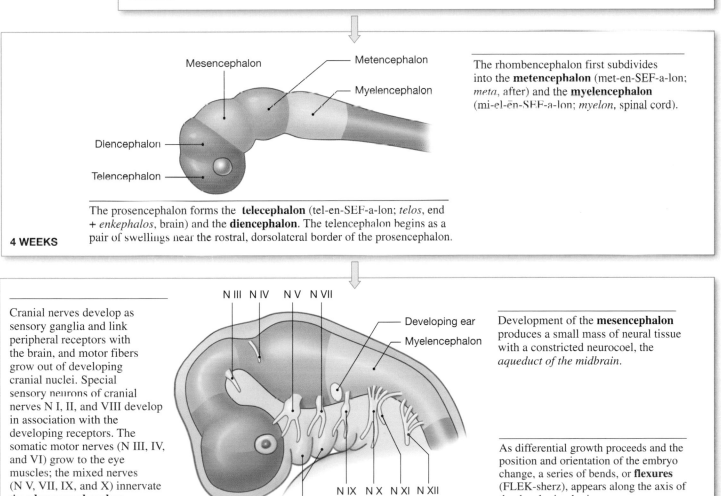

N III N IV   N V N VII

Developing ear

Myelencephalon

N IX N X N XI N XII

Pharyngeal arches

Development of the **mesencephalon** produces a small mass of neural tissue with a constricted neurocoel, the *aqueduct of the midbrain*.

As differential growth proceeds and the position and orientation of the embryo change, a series of bends, or **flexures** (FLEK-sherz), appears along the axis of the developing brain.

5 WEEKS

EMBRYOLOGY SUMMARY   12: THE DEVELOPMENT OF THE BRAIN AND CRANIAL NERVES—*PART I*

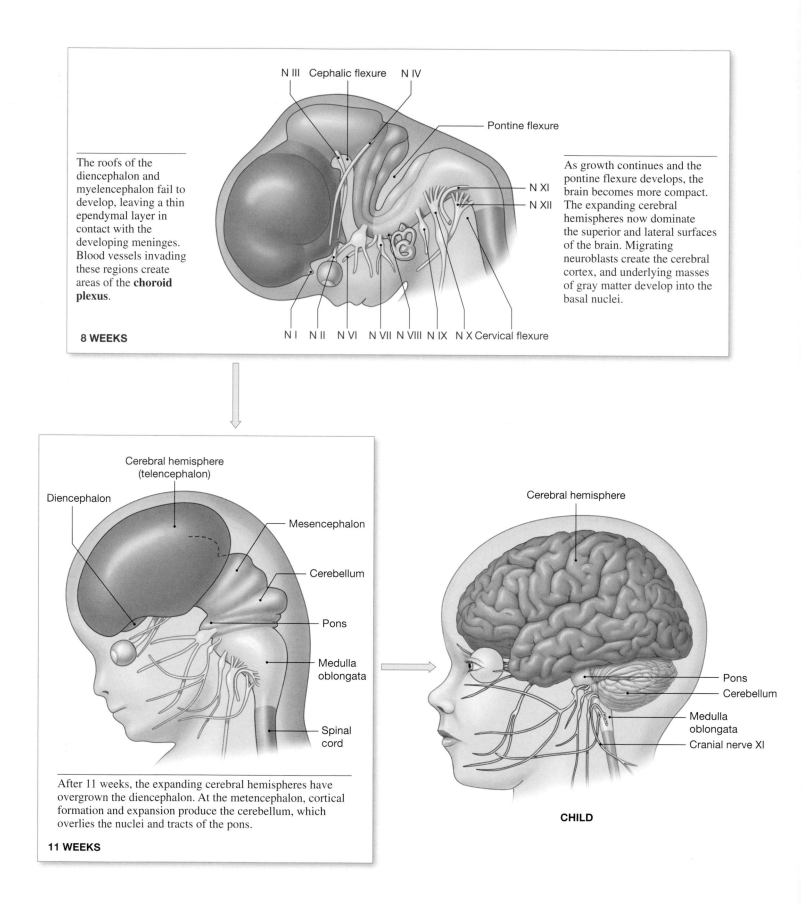

N III Cephalic flexure N IV

Pontine flexure

The roofs of the diencephalon and myelencephalon fail to develop, leaving a thin ependymal layer in contact with the developing meninges. Blood vessels invading these regions create areas of the **choroid plexus**.

N XI
N XII

As growth continues and the pontine flexure develops, the brain becomes more compact. The expanding cerebral hemispheres now dominate the superior and lateral surfaces of the brain. Migrating neuroblasts create the cerebral cortex, and underlying masses of gray matter develop into the basal nuclei.

8 WEEKS

N I   N II   N VI   N VII N VIII N IX N X Cervical flexure

Cerebral hemisphere (telencephalon)

Diencephalon

Mesencephalon

Cerebellum

Pons

Medulla oblongata

Spinal cord

After 11 weeks, the expanding cerebral hemispheres have overgrown the diencephalon. At the metencephalon, cortical formation and expansion produce the cerebellum, which overlies the nuclei and tracts of the pons.

11 WEEKS

Cerebral hemisphere

Pons
Cerebellum

Medulla oblongata

Cranial nerve XI

CHILD

EMBRYOLOGY SUMMARY **12:** THE DEVELOPMENT OF THE BRAIN AND CRANIAL NERVES—*PART II*

All special sense organs develop from the interaction between the epithelia and the developing nervous system of the embryo.

VISION

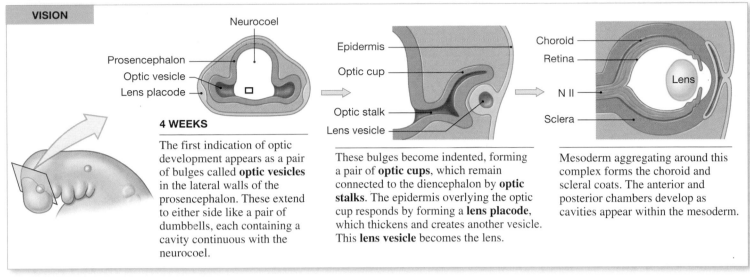

4 WEEKS

The first indication of optic development appears as a pair of bulges called **optic vesicles** in the lateral walls of the prosencephalon. These extend to either side like a pair of dumbbells, each containing a cavity continuous with the neurocoel.

These bulges become indented, forming a pair of **optic cups**, which remain connected to the diencephalon by **optic stalks**. The epidermis overlying the optic cup responds by forming a **lens placode**, which thickens and creates another vesicle. This **lens vesicle** becomes the lens.

Mesoderm aggregating around this complex forms the choroid and scleral coats. The anterior and posterior chambers develop as cavities appear within the mesoderm.

OLFACTION

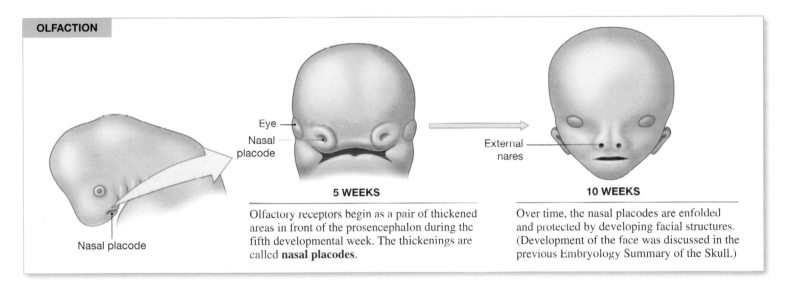

5 WEEKS

Olfactory receptors begin as a pair of thickened areas in front of the prosencephalon during the fifth developmental week. The thickenings are called **nasal placodes**.

10 WEEKS

Over time, the nasal placodes are enfolded and protected by developing facial structures. (Development of the face was discussed in the previous Embryology Summary of the Skull.)

GUSTATION

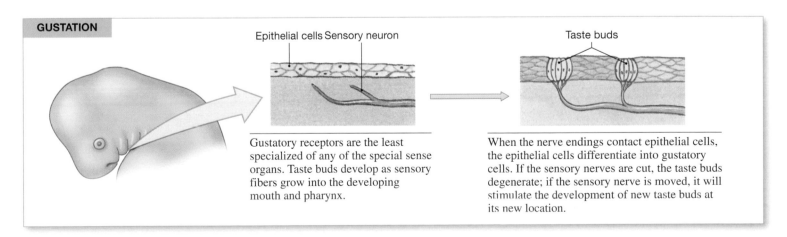

Gustatory receptors are the least specialized of any of the special sense organs. Taste buds develop as sensory fibers grow into the developing mouth and pharynx.

When the nerve endings contact epithelial cells, the epithelial cells differentiate into gustatory cells. If the sensory nerves are cut, the taste buds degenerate; if the sensory nerve is moved, it will stimulate the development of new taste buds at its new location.

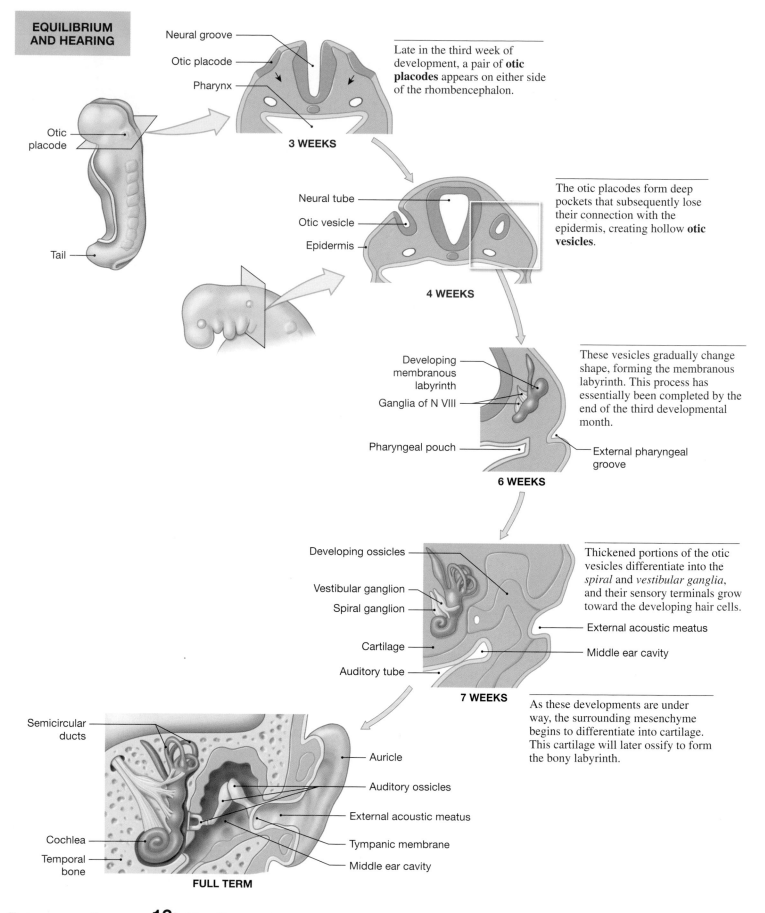

EQUILIBRIUM AND HEARING

Otic placode

Tail

Neural groove

Otic placode

Pharynx

3 WEEKS

Late in the third week of development, a pair of **otic placodes** appears on either side of the rhombencephalon.

Neural tube

Otic vesicle

Epidermis

4 WEEKS

The otic placodes form deep pockets that subsequently lose their connection with the epidermis, creating hollow **otic vesicles**.

Developing membranous labyrinth

Ganglia of N VIII

Pharyngeal pouch

External pharyngeal groove

6 WEEKS

These vesicles gradually change shape, forming the membranous labyrinth. This process has essentially been completed by the end of the third developmental month.

Developing ossicles

Vestibular ganglion

Spiral ganglion

Cartilage

Auditory tube

External acoustic meatus

Middle ear cavity

7 WEEKS

Thickened portions of the otic vesicles differentiate into the *spiral* and *vestibular ganglia*, and their sensory terminals grow toward the developing hair cells.

Semicircular ducts

Cochlea

Temporal bone

Auricle

Auditory ossicles

External acoustic meatus

Tympanic membrane

Middle ear cavity

FULL TERM

As these developments are under way, the surrounding mesenchyme begins to differentiate into cartilage. This cartilage will later ossify to form the bony labyrinth.

EMBRYOLOGY SUMMARY 13: THE DEVELOPMENT OF SPECIAL SENSE ORGANS—PART II

As noted in Chapter 4, all secretory glands, whether exocrine or endocrine, are derived from epithelia. Endocrine organs develop from epithelia (1) covering the outside of the embryo, (2) lining the digestive tract, and (3) lining the coelomic cavity.

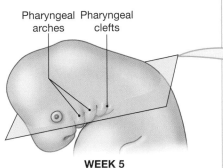

WEEK 5

The pharyngeal region of the embryo plays a particularly important role in endocrine development. After 4–5 weeks of development, the *pharyngeal arches* are well formed. Human embryos develop five or six pharyngeal arches, not all visible from the exterior. (Arch 5 may not appear or may form and degenerate almost immediately.) The five major arches (I–IV, VI) are separated by *pharyngeal clefts*, deep ectodermal grooves.

PARATHYROID GLANDS AND THYMUS

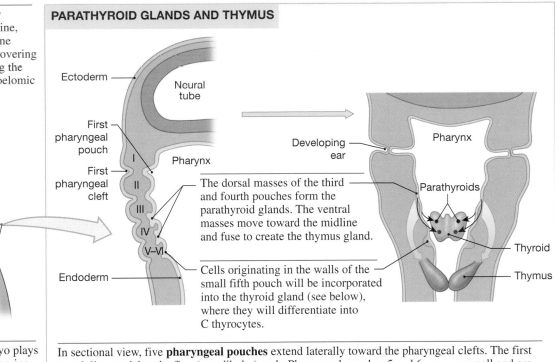

The dorsal masses of the third and fourth pouches form the parathyroid glands. The ventral masses move toward the midline and fuse to create the thymus gland.

Cells originating in the walls of the small fifth pouch will be incorporated into the thyroid gland (see below), where they will differentiate into C thyrocytes.

In sectional view, five **pharyngeal pouches** extend laterally toward the pharyngeal clefts. The first pouch lies caudal to the first (mandibular) arch. Pharyngeal pouches 5 and 6 are very small and are interconnected. Endoderm lining the third, fourth, and fifth pairs of pharyngeal pouches forms dorsal and ventral masses of cells that migrate beneath the endodermal epithelium.

THYROID GLAND

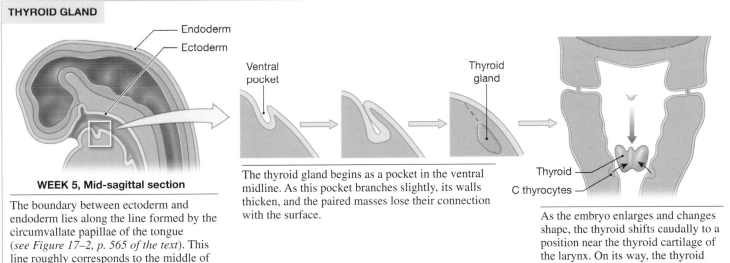

WEEK 5, Mid-sagittal section

The boundary between ectoderm and endoderm lies along the line formed by the circumvallate papillae of the tongue (*see Figure 17–2, p. 565 of the text*). This line roughly corresponds to the middle of the mandibular (first) arch. The thyroid gland forms here in the ventral midline.

The thyroid gland begins as a pocket in the ventral midline. As this pocket branches slightly, its walls thicken, and the paired masses lose their connection with the surface.

As the embryo enlarges and changes shape, the thyroid shifts caudally to a position near the thyroid cartilage of the larynx. On its way, the thyroid gland incorporates C thyrocytes from the walls of the fifth pouch.

PITUITARY GLAND

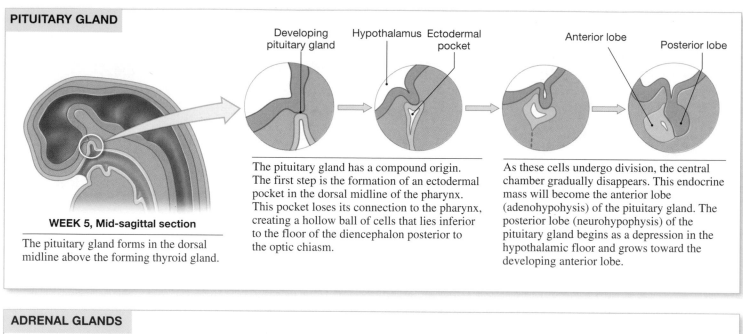

WEEK 5, Mid-sagittal section

The pituitary gland forms in the dorsal midline above the forming thyroid gland.

The pituitary gland has a compound origin. The first step is the formation of an ectodermal pocket in the dorsal midline of the pharynx. This pocket loses its connection to the pharynx, creating a hollow ball of cells that lies inferior to the floor of the diencephalon posterior to the optic chiasm.

As these cells undergo division, the central chamber gradually disappears. This endocrine mass will become the anterior lobe (adenohypophysis) of the pituitary gland. The posterior lobe (neurohypophysis) of the pituitary gland begins as a depression in the hypothalamic floor and grows toward the developing anterior lobe.

ADRENAL GLANDS

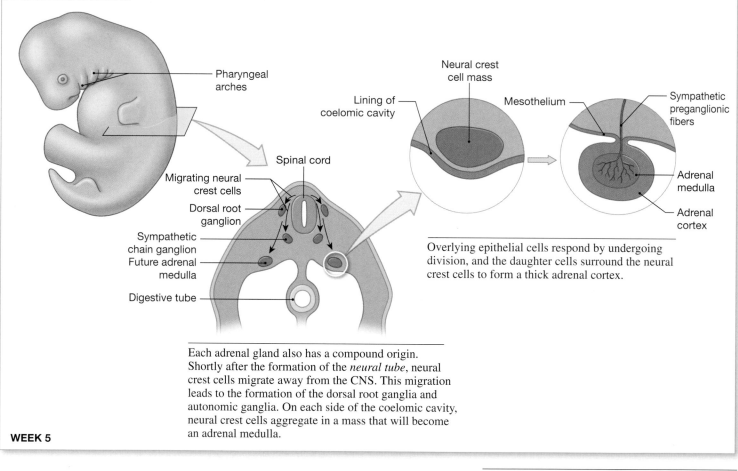

Each adrenal gland also has a compound origin. Shortly after the formation of the *neural tube*, neural crest cells migrate away from the CNS. This migration leads to the formation of the dorsal root ganglia and autonomic ganglia. On each side of the coelomic cavity, neural crest cells aggregate in a mass that will become an adrenal medulla.

Overlying epithelial cells respond by undergoing division, and the daughter cells surround the neural crest cells to form a thick adrenal cortex.

WEEK 5

For additional details concerning the development of other endocrine organs, refer to the subsequent Embryology Summaries on the Lymphatic, Digestive, Urinary, and Reproductive systems.

EMBRYOLOGY SUMMARY **14:** THE DEVELOPMENT OF THE ENDOCRINE SYSTEM—*PART II*

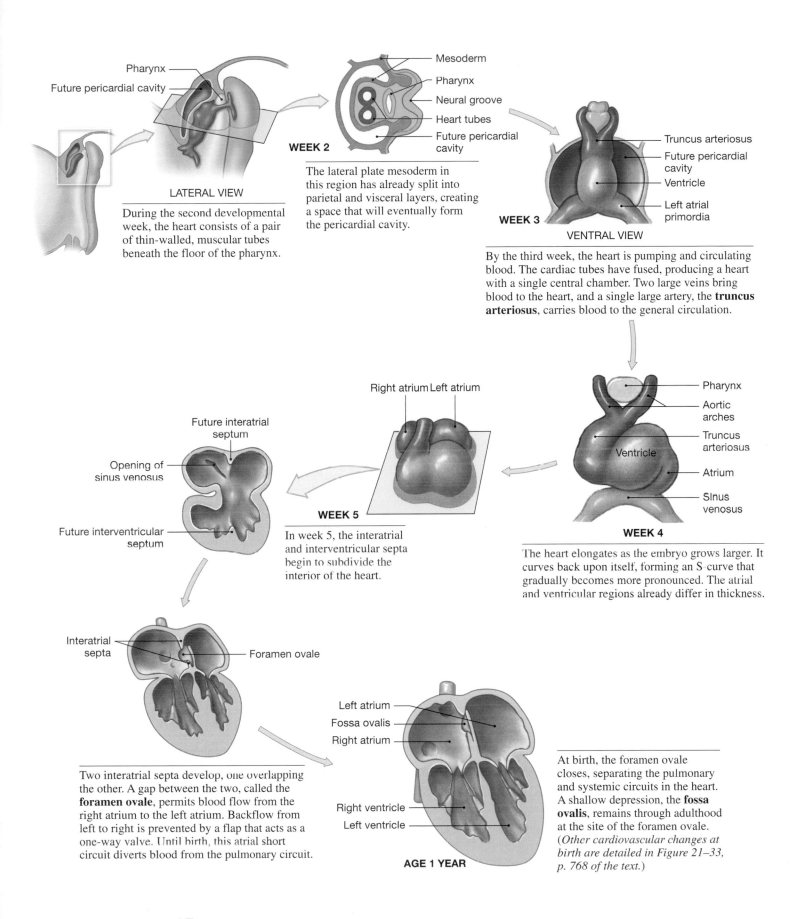

Pharynx
Future pericardial cavity

LATERAL VIEW

During the second developmental week, the heart consists of a pair of thin-walled, muscular tubes beneath the floor of the pharynx.

Mesoderm
Pharynx
Neural groove
Heart tubes
Future pericardial cavity

WEEK 2

The lateral plate mesoderm in this region has already split into parietal and visceral layers, creating a space that will eventually form the pericardial cavity.

Truncus arteriosus
Future pericardial cavity
Ventricle
Left atrial primordia

WEEK 3
VENTRAL VIEW

By the third week, the heart is pumping and circulating blood. The cardiac tubes have fused, producing a heart with a single central chamber. Two large veins bring blood to the heart, and a single large artery, the **truncus arteriosus**, carries blood to the general circulation.

Right atrium **Left atrium**

Future interatrial septum

Opening of sinus venosus

Future interventricular septum

WEEK 5

In week 5, the interatrial and interventricular septa begin to subdivide the interior of the heart.

Pharynx
Aortic arches
Truncus arteriosus
Ventricle
Atrium
Sinus venosus

WEEK 4

The heart elongates as the embryo grows larger. It curves back upon itself, forming an S-curve that gradually becomes more pronounced. The atrial and ventricular regions already differ in thickness.

Interatrial septa
Foramen ovale

Two interatrial septa develop, one overlapping the other. A gap between the two, called the **foramen ovale**, permits blood flow from the right atrium to the left atrium. Backflow from left to right is prevented by a flap that acts as a one-way valve. Until birth, this atrial short circuit diverts blood from the pulmonary circuit.

Left atrium
Fossa ovalis
Right atrium
Right ventricle
Left ventricle

AGE 1 YEAR

At birth, the foramen ovale closes, separating the pulmonary and systemic circuits in the heart. A shallow depression, the **fossa ovalis**, remains through adulthood at the site of the foramen ovale. (*Other cardiovascular changes at birth are detailed in Figure 21–33, p. 768 of the text.*)

EMBRYOLOGY SUMMARY 15: THE DEVELOPMENT OF THE HEART

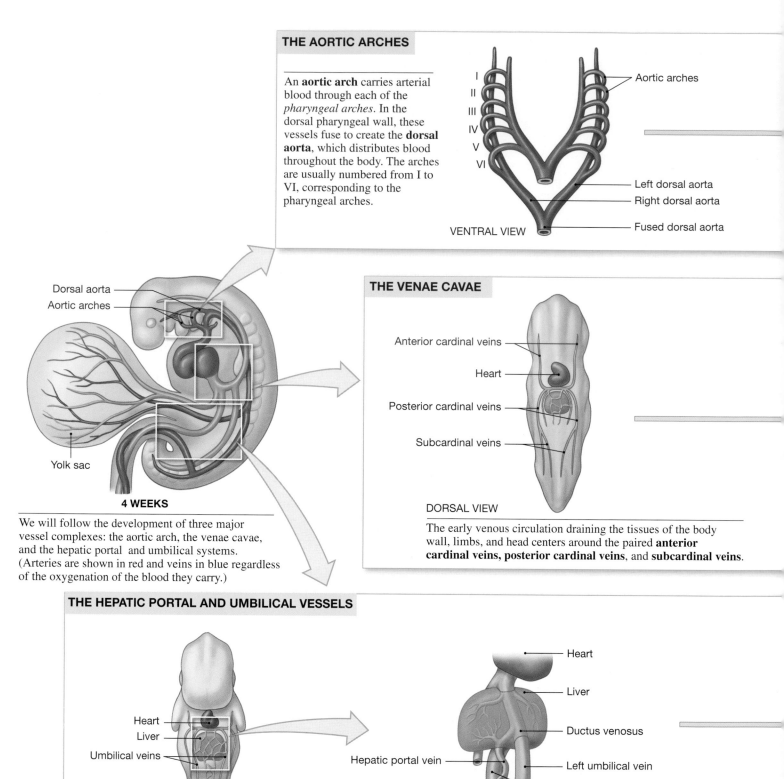

THE AORTIC ARCHES

An **aortic arch** carries arterial blood through each of the *pharyngeal arches*. In the dorsal pharyngeal wall, these vessels fuse to create the **dorsal aorta**, which distributes blood throughout the body. The arches are usually numbered from I to VI, corresponding to the pharyngeal arches.

I
II
III
IV
V
VI

Aortic arches

Left dorsal aorta

Right dorsal aorta

Fused dorsal aorta

VENTRAL VIEW

Dorsal aorta
Aortic arches

Yolk sac

4 WEEKS

We will follow the development of three major vessel complexes: the aortic arch, the venae cavae, and the hepatic portal and umbilical systems. (Arteries are shown in red and veins in blue regardless of the oxygenation of the blood they carry.)

THE VENAE CAVAE

Anterior cardinal veins

Heart

Posterior cardinal veins

Subcardinal veins

DORSAL VIEW

The early venous circulation draining the tissues of the body wall, limbs, and head centers around the paired **anterior cardinal veins, posterior cardinal veins**, and **subcardinal veins**.

THE HEPATIC PORTAL AND UMBILICAL VESSELS

Heart
Liver
Umbilical veins

Umbilical arteries

4 WEEKS

Paired **umbilical arteries** deliver blood to the placenta. At 4 weeks, paired **umbilical veins** return blood to capillary networks in the liver. Veins running along the length of the digestive tract have extensive interconnections.

Heart

Liver

Ductus venosus

Hepatic portal vein

Left umbilical vein

Right umbilical vein

Digestive tract

12 WEEKS

By week 12, the right umbilical vein disintegrates, and the blood from the placenta travels along a single umbilical vein. The **ductus venosus** allows some venous blood to bypass the liver. The veins draining the digestive tract have fused, forming the hepatic portal vein.

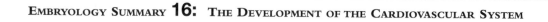

EMBRYOLOGY SUMMARY 16: THE DEVELOPMENT OF THE CARDIOVASCULAR SYSTEM

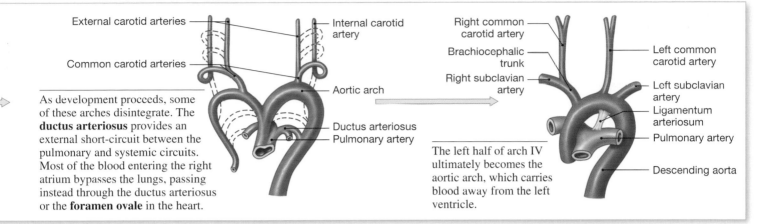

External carotid arteries

Internal carotid artery

Common carotid arteries

Aortic arch

Ductus arteriosus

Pulmonary artery

As development proceeds, some of these arches disintegrate. The **ductus arteriosus** provides an external short-circuit between the pulmonary and systemic circuits. Most of the blood entering the right atrium bypasses the lungs, passing instead through the ductus arteriosus or the **foramen ovale** in the heart.

Right common carotid artery

Brachiocephalic trunk

Right subclavian artery

Left common carotid artery

Left subclavian artery

Ligamentum arteriosum

Pulmonary artery

Descending aorta

The left half of arch IV ultimately becomes the aortic arch, which carries blood away from the left ventricle.

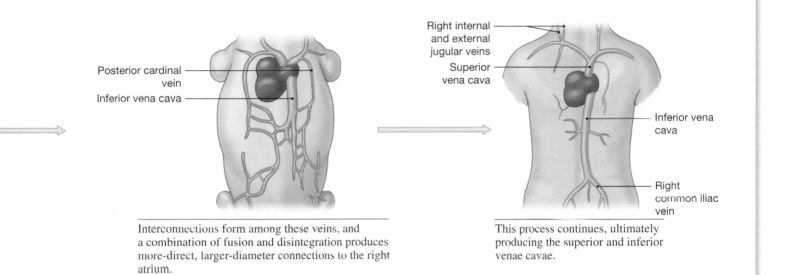

Posterior cardinal vein

Inferior vena cava

Right internal and external jugular veins

Superior vena cava

Inferior vena cava

Right common iliac vein

Interconnections form among these veins, and a combination of fusion and disintegration produces more-direct, larger-diameter connections to the right atrium.

This process continues, ultimately producing the superior and inferior venae cavae.

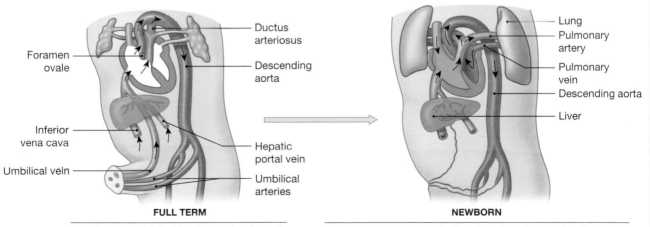

Foramen ovale

Ductus arteriosus

Descending aorta

Inferior vena cava

Umbilical vein

Hepatic portal vein

Umbilical arteries

FULL TERM

Lung

Pulmonary artery

Pulmonary vein

Descending aorta

Liver

NEWBORN

Shortly before birth, blood returning from the placenta travels through the liver in the ductus venosus to reach the inferior vena cava. Much of the blood delivered by the venae cavae bypasses the lungs by traveling through the foramen ovale and the ductus arteriosus.

At birth, pressures drop in the pleural cavities as the chest expands and the infant takes its first breath. The pulmonary vessels dilate, and blood flow to the lungs increases. Pressure falls in the right atrium, and the higher left atrial pressures close the valve that guards the foramen ovale. Smooth muscles contract the ductus arteriosus, which ultimately converts to the **ligamentum arteriosum**, a fibrous strand.

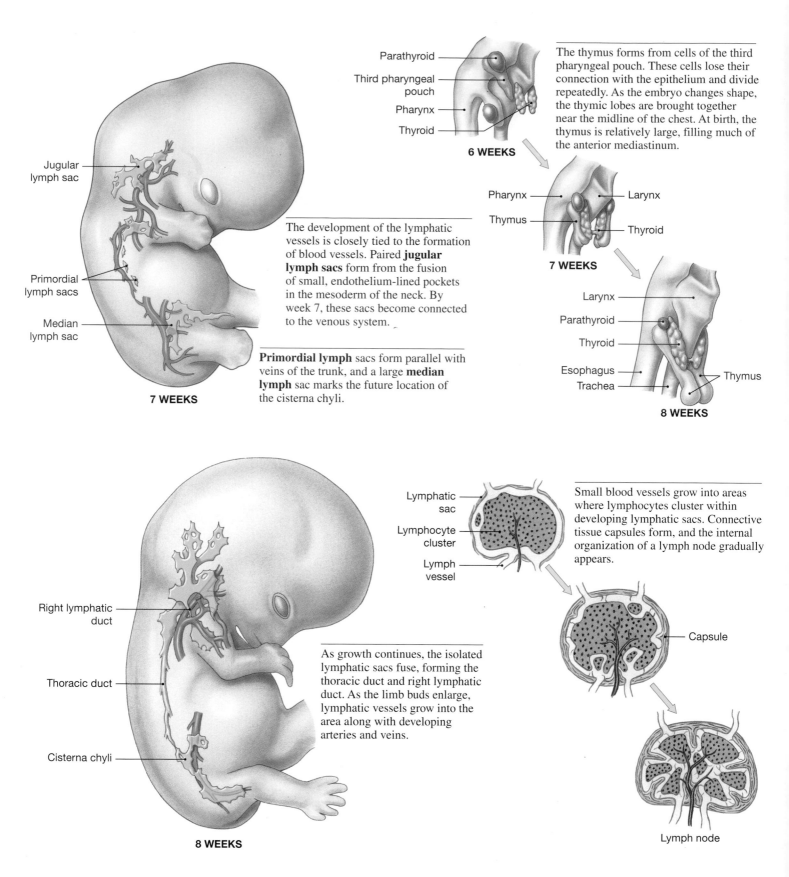

Parathyroid

Third pharyngeal pouch

Pharynx

Thyroid

6 WEEKS

The thymus forms from cells of the third pharyngeal pouch. These cells lose their connection with the epithelium and divide repeatedly. As the embryo changes shape, the thymic lobes are brought together near the midline of the chest. At birth, the thymus is relatively large, filling much of the anterior mediastinum.

Pharynx

Larynx

Thymus

Thyroid

7 WEEKS

Larynx

Parathyroid

Thyroid

Esophagus

Trachea

Thymus

8 WEEKS

Jugular lymph sac

Primordial lymph sacs

Median lymph sac

7 WEEKS

The development of the lymphatic vessels is closely tied to the formation of blood vessels. Paired **jugular lymph sacs** form from the fusion of small, endothelium-lined pockets in the mesoderm of the neck. By week 7, these sacs become connected to the venous system.

Primordial lymph sacs form parallel with veins of the trunk, and a large **median lymph** sac marks the future location of the cisterna chyli.

Right lymphatic duct

Thoracic duct

Cisterna chyli

8 WEEKS

As growth continues, the isolated lymphatic sacs fuse, forming the thoracic duct and right lymphatic duct. As the limb buds enlarge, lymphatic vessels grow into the area along with developing arteries and veins.

Lymphatic sac

Lymphocyte cluster

Lymph vessel

Small blood vessels grow into areas where lymphocytes cluster within developing lymphatic sacs. Connective tissue capsules form, and the internal organization of a lymph node gradually appears.

Capsule

Lymph node

EMBRYOLOGY SUMMARY **17:** THE DEVELOPMENT OF THE LYMPHATIC SYSTEM

THE LUNGS

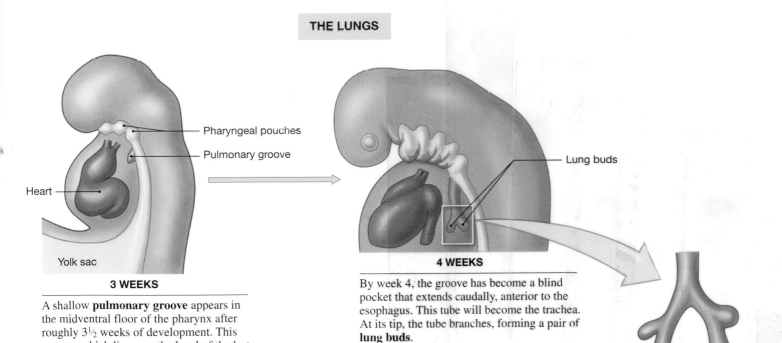

Heart

Pharyngeal pouches

Pulmonary groove

Yolk sac

3 WEEKS

A shallow **pulmonary groove** appears in the midventral floor of the pharynx after roughly 3½ weeks of development. This groove, which lies near the level of the last pharyngeal arch, gradually deepens.

Lung buds

4 WEEKS

By week 4, the groove has become a blind pocket that extends caudally, anterior to the esophagus. This tube will become the trachea. At its tip, the tube branches, forming a pair of **lung buds**.

The lung buds continue to elongate and branch repeatedly.

3 MONTHS

By the end of the sixth fetal month, there are around a million terminal branches, and the conducting passageways are complete to the level of the bronchioles.

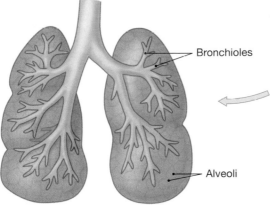

Bronchioles

Alveoli

Over the next three months, each of the bronchioles gives rise to several hundred alveoli. This process continues for a variable period after birth.

THE PLEURAL CAVITIES

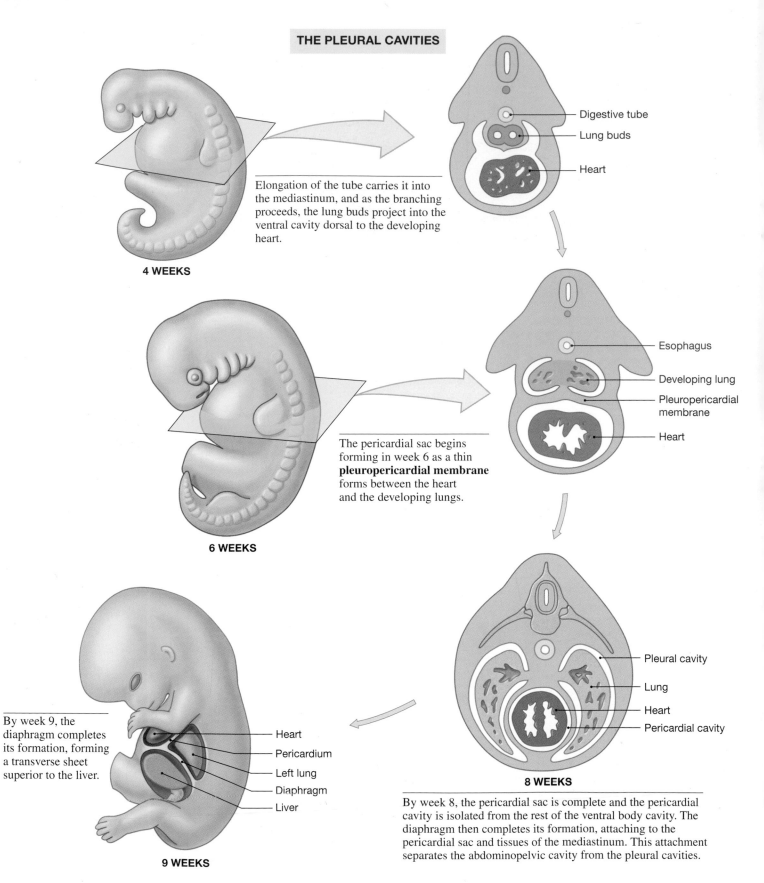

4 WEEKS

— Digestive tube

— Lung buds

— Heart

Elongation of the tube carries it into the mediastinum, and as the branching proceeds, the lung buds project into the ventral cavity dorsal to the developing heart.

6 WEEKS

— Esophagus

— Developing lung

— Pleuropericardial membrane

— Heart

The pericardial sac begins forming in week 6 as a thin **pleuropericardial membrane** forms between the heart and the developing lungs.

— Pleural cavity

— Lung

— Heart

— Pericardial cavity

8 WEEKS

By week 8, the pericardial sac is complete and the pericardial cavity is isolated from the rest of the ventral body cavity. The diaphragm then completes its formation, attaching to the pericardial sac and tissues of the mediastinum. This attachment separates the abdominopelvic cavity from the pleural cavities.

By week 9, the diaphragm completes its formation, forming a transverse sheet superior to the liver.

— Heart

— Pericardium

— Left lung

— Diaphragm

— Liver

9 WEEKS

EMBRYOLOGY SUMMARY **18:** THE DEVELOPMENT OF THE RESPIRATORY SYSTEM—*PART II*

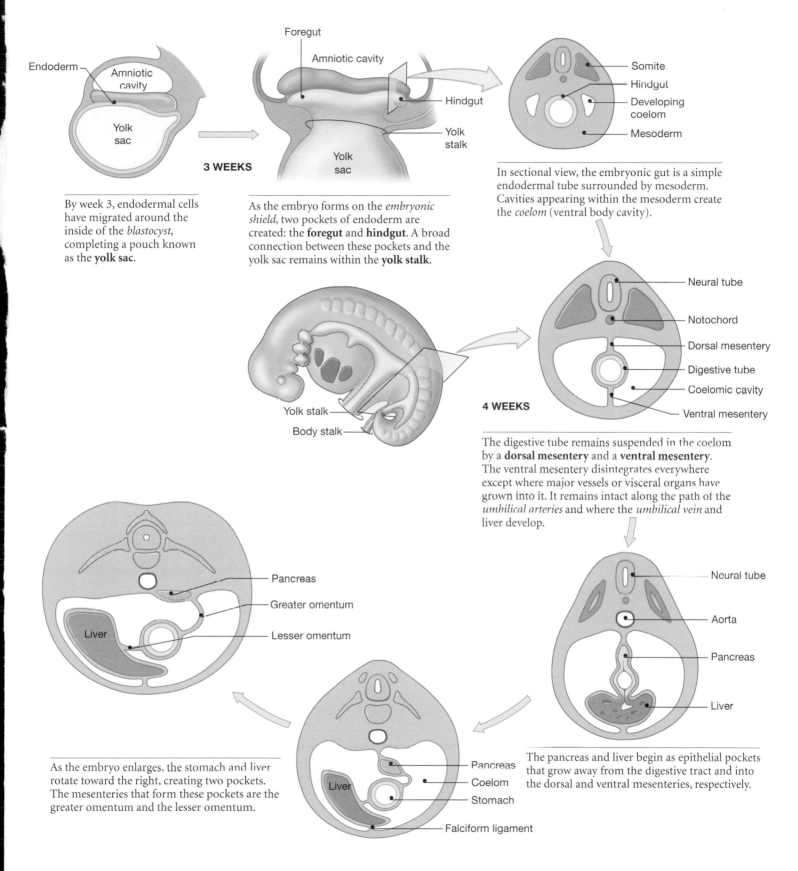

3 WEEKS

By week 3, endodermal cells have migrated around the inside of the *blastocyst*, completing a pouch known as the **yolk sac**.

As the embryo forms on the *embryonic shield*, two pockets of endoderm are created: the **foregut** and **hindgut**. A broad connection between these pockets and the yolk sac remains within the **yolk stalk**.

In sectional view, the embryonic gut is a simple endodermal tube surrounded by mesoderm. Cavities appearing within the mesoderm create the *coelom* (ventral body cavity).

4 WEEKS

The digestive tube remains suspended in the coelom by a **dorsal mesentery** and a **ventral mesentery**. The ventral mesentery disintegrates everywhere except where major vessels or visceral organs have grown into it. It remains intact along the path of the *umbilical arteries* and where the *umbilical vein* and liver develop.

As the embryo enlarges, the stomach and liver rotate toward the right, creating two pockets. The mesenteries that form these pockets are the greater omentum and the lesser omentum.

The pancreas and liver begin as epithelial pockets that grow away from the digestive tract and into the dorsal and ventral mesenteries, respectively.

EMBRYOLOGY SUMMARY 19: THE DEVELOPMENT OF THE DIGESTIVE SYSTEM—PART I

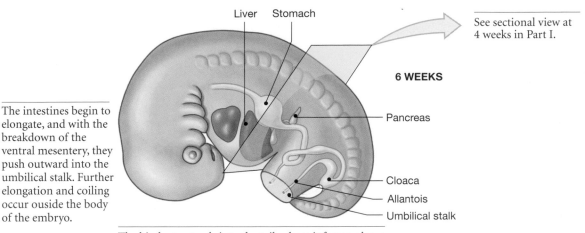

See sectional view at 4 weeks in Part I.

6 WEEKS

The intestines begin to elongate, and with the breakdown of the ventral mesentery, they push outward into the umbilical stalk. Further elongation and coiling occur ouside the body of the embryo.

Liver   Stomach

Pancreas

Cloaca

Allantois

Umbilical stalk

The hindgut extends into the tail, where it forms a large chamber, the **cloaca**. A tubular extension of the cloaca, the **allantois** (a-LAN-tō-is; *allantos*, sausage) projects away from the body and into the **body stalk**. Fusion of the yolk stalk and body stalk will create the **umbilical stalk**, also known as the *umbilical cord*.

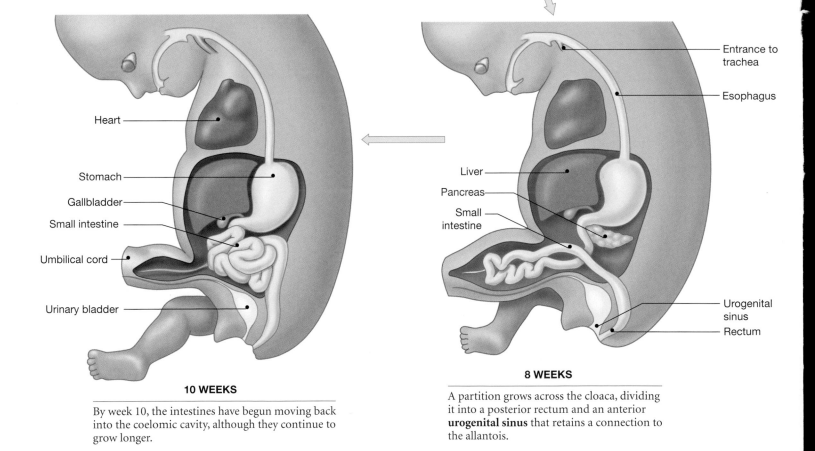

Heart

Stomach

Gallbladder

Small intestine

Umbilical cord

Urinary bladder

10 WEEKS

By week 10, the intestines have begun moving back into the coelomic cavity, although they continue to grow longer.

Entrance to trachea

Esophagus

Liver

Pancreas

Small intestine

Urogenital sinus

Rectum

8 WEEKS

A partition grows across the cloaca, dividing it into a posterior rectum and an anterior **urogenital sinus** that retains a connection to the allantois.

EMBRYOLOGY SUMMARY **19:** THE DEVELOPMENT OF THE DIGESTIVE SYSTEM—*PART II*

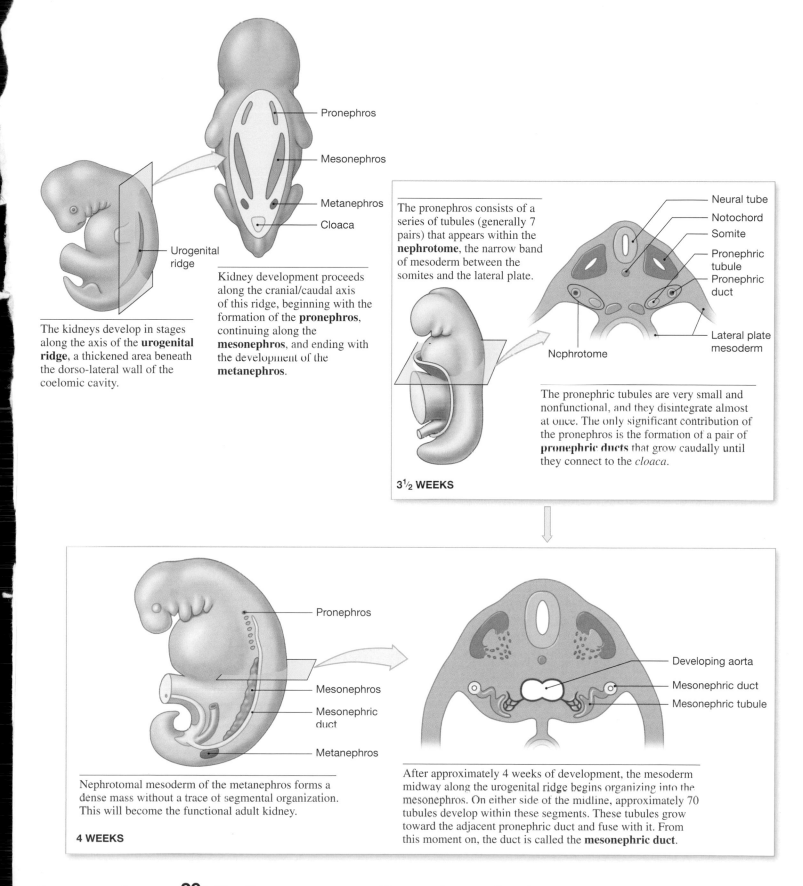

Pronephros

Mesonephros

Metanephros

Cloaca

Urogenital ridge

The kidneys develop in stages along the axis of the **urogenital ridge**, a thickened area beneath the dorso-lateral wall of the coelomic cavity.

Kidney development proceeds along the cranial/caudal axis of this ridge, beginning with the formation of the **pronephros**, continuing along the **mesonephros**, and ending with the development of the **metanephros**.

The pronephros consists of a series of tubules (generally 7 pairs) that appears within the **nephrotome**, the narrow band of mesoderm between the somites and the lateral plate.

Neural tube

Notochord

Somite

Pronephric tubule

Pronephric duct

Lateral plate mesoderm

Nephrotome

The pronephric tubules are very small and nonfunctional, and they disintegrate almost at once. The only significant contribution of the pronephros is the formation of a pair of **pronephric ducts** that grow caudally until they connect to the *cloaca*.

3¹/₂ WEEKS

Pronephros

Mesonephros

Mesonephric duct

Metanephros

Developing aorta

Mesonephric duct

Mesonephric tubule

Nephrotomal mesoderm of the metanephros forms a dense mass without a trace of segmental organization. This will become the functional adult kidney.

4 WEEKS

After approximately 4 weeks of development, the mesoderm midway along the urogenital ridge begins organizing into the mesonephros. On either side of the midline, approximately 70 tubules develop within these segments. These tubules grow toward the adjacent pronephric duct and fuse with it. From this moment on, the duct is called the **mesonephric duct**.

EMBRYOLOGY SUMMARY 20: **THE DEVELOPMENT OF THE URINARY SYSTEM—PART I**

A **ureteric bud**, or *metanephric diverticulum*, forms in the wall of each mesonephric duct, and this blind tube elongates and branches within the adjacent metanephros. Tubules developing within the metanephros then connect to the terminal branch of the ureteric bud.

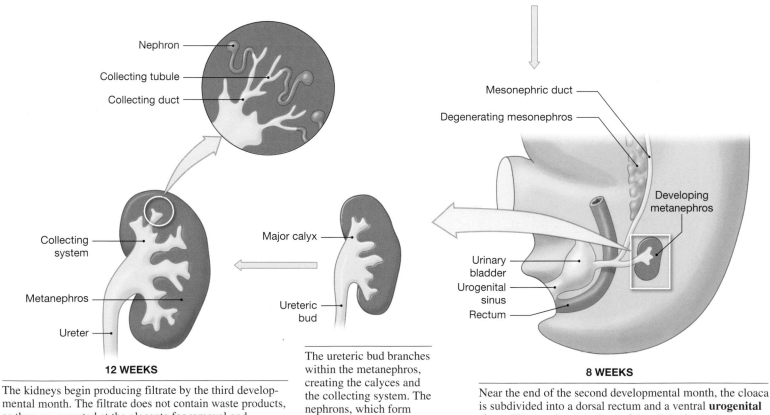

Mesonephros
Allantois
Mesonephric duct
Cloaca
Ureteric bud
Metanephros

Glomerulus
Mesonephric duct
Renal corpuscle

In each segment, a branch of the aorta grows toward the nephrotome, and the tubules form large nephrons with enormous glomeruli. Like the pronephros, the mesonephros does not persist, and when the last segments of the mesonephros are forming, the first are already beginning to degenerate.

Most of the metabolic wastes produced by the developing embryo are passed across the placenta to enter the maternal circulation. The small amount of urine produced by the kidneys accumulates within the cloaca and the *allantois*, an endoderm-lined sac that extends into the umbilical stalk.

6 WEEKS

Nephron
Collecting tubule
Collecting duct

Mesonephric duct
Degenerating mesonephros

Collecting system

Major calyx

Developing metanephros

Metanephros

Urinary bladder
Urogenital sinus
Rectum

Ureter

Ureteric bud

12 WEEKS

The kidneys begin producing filtrate by the third developmental month. The filtrate does not contain waste products, as they are excreted at the placenta for removal and elimination by the maternal kidneys. The sterile filtrate mixes with the amniotic fluid and is swallowed by the fetus and reabsorbed across the lining of the digestive tract.

The ureteric bud branches within the metanephros, creating the calyces and the collecting system. The nephrons, which form within the mesoderm of the metanephros, tap into the collecting tubules.

8 WEEKS

Near the end of the second developmental month, the cloaca is subdivided into a dorsal rectum and a ventral **urogenital sinus**. The proximal portions of the allantois persist as the **urinary bladder**, and the connection between the bladder and an opening on the body surface will form the **urethra**.

EMBRYOLOGY SUMMARY 20: THE DEVELOPMENT OF THE URINARY SYSTEM—PART II

SEXUALLY INDIFFERENT STAGES
(WEEKS 3–6)

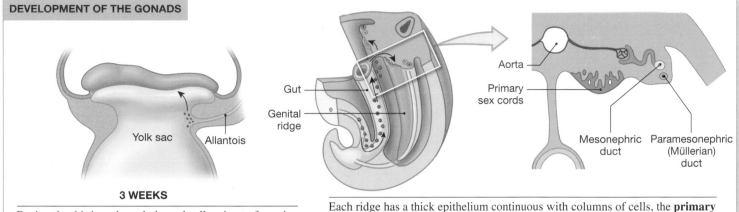

DEVELOPMENT OF THE GONADS

3 WEEKS

During the third week, endodermal cells migrate from the wall of the yolk sac near the allantois to the dorsal wall of the abdominal cavity. These primordial germ cells enter the **genital ridges** that parallel the mesonephros.

Each ridge has a thick epithelium continuous with columns of cells, the **primary sex cords**, that extend into the center (medulla) of the ridge. Anterior to each mesonephric duct, a duct forms that has no connection to the kidneys. This is the **paramesonephric** (*Müllerian*) **duct**; it extends along the genital ridge and continues toward the cloaca. At this sexually indifferent stage, male embryos cannot be distinguished from female embryos.

DEVELOPMENT OF DUCTS AND ACCESSORY ORGANS

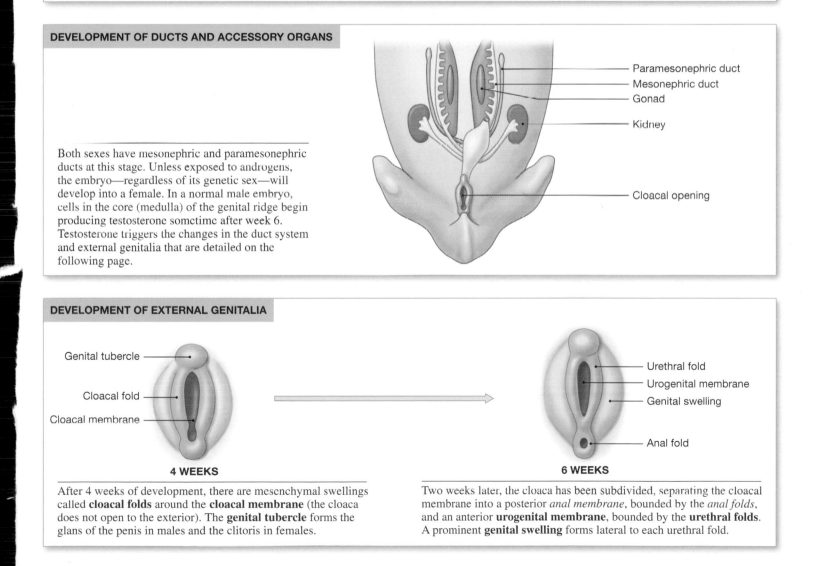

Both sexes have mesonephric and paramesonephric ducts at this stage. Unless exposed to androgens, the embryo—regardless of its genetic sex—will develop into a female. In a normal male embryo, cells in the core (medulla) of the genital ridge begin producing testosterone sometime after week 6. Testosterone triggers the changes in the duct system and external genitalia that are detailed on the following page.

DEVELOPMENT OF EXTERNAL GENITALIA

4 WEEKS

After 4 weeks of development, there are mesenchymal swellings called **cloacal folds** around the **cloacal membrane** (the cloaca does not open to the exterior). The **genital tubercle** forms the glans of the penis in males and the clitoris in females.

6 WEEKS

Two weeks later, the cloaca has been subdivided, separating the cloacal membrane into a posterior *anal membrane*, bounded by the *anal folds*, and an anterior **urogenital membrane**, bounded by the **urethral folds**. A prominent **genital swelling** forms lateral to each urethral fold.

EMBRYOLOGY SUMMARY **21:** THE DEVELOPMENT OF THE REPRODUCTIVE SYSTEM—*PART I*

DEVELOPMENT OF THE MALE REPRODUCTIVE SYSTEM

DEVELOPMENT OF THE TESTES

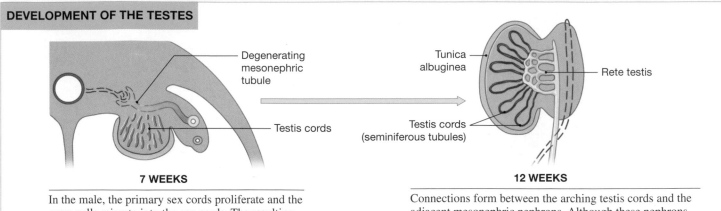

7 WEEKS

In the male, the primary sex cords proliferate and the germ cells migrate into the sex cords. The resulting **testis cords** will form the seminiferous tubules.

12 WEEKS

Connections form between the arching testis cords and the adjacent mesonephric nephrons. Although these nephrons later degenerate, the seminiferous tubules remain connected to the mesonephric duct.

DEVELOPMENT OF MALE DUCTS AND ACCESSORY ORGANS

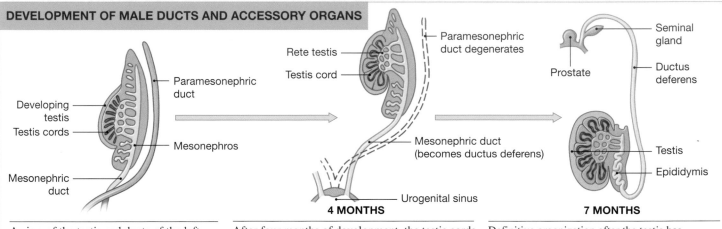

4 MONTHS

7 MONTHS

A view of the testis and ducts of the left side as seen in frontal section. Note the location and orientation of the mesonephros relative to the developing testis.

After four months of development, the testis cords are connected to the remnants of the mesonephric tubules by the rete testis. The paramesonephric (Müllerian) duct has degenerated.

Definitive organization after the testis has descended into the scrotum (*see Figure 28–2, p. 1044*). Note the relationships between the definitive sex organs and the embryonic structures.

DEVELOPMENT OF MALE EXTERNAL GENITALIA

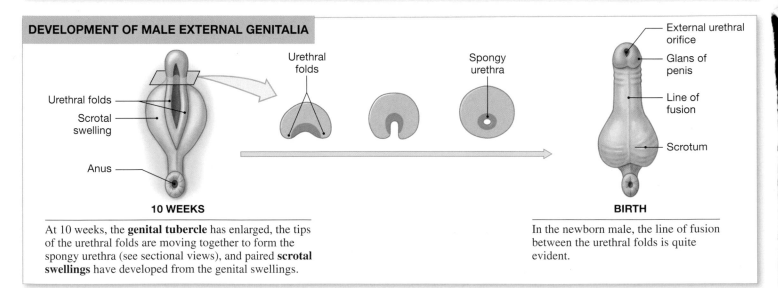

10 WEEKS

At 10 weeks, the **genital tubercle** has enlarged, the tips of the urethral folds are moving together to form the spongy urethra (see sectional views), and paired **scrotal swellings** have developed from the genital swellings.

BIRTH

In the newborn male, the line of fusion between the urethral folds is quite evident.

DEVELOPMENT OF THE FEMALE REPRODUCTIVE SYSTEM

DEVELOPMENT OF THE OVARIES

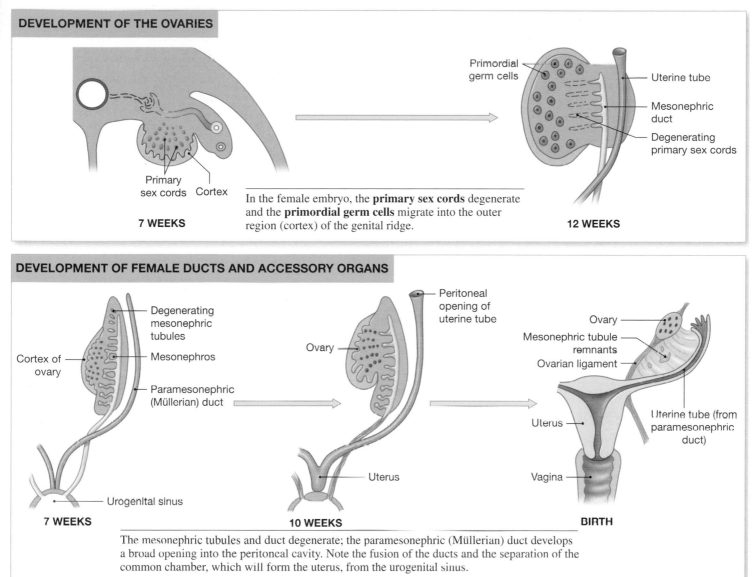

In the female embryo, the **primary sex cords** degenerate and the **primordial germ cells** migrate into the outer region (cortex) of the genital ridge.

DEVELOPMENT OF FEMALE DUCTS AND ACCESSORY ORGANS

The mesonephric tubules and duct degenerate; the paramesonephric (Müllerian) duct develops a broad opening into the peritoneal cavity. Note the fusion of the ducts and the separation of the common chamber, which will form the uterus, from the urogenital sinus.

COMPARISON OF MALE AND FEMALE EXTERNAL GENITALIA

Males	Females
Penis	Clitoris
Corpora cavernosa	Erectile tissue
Corpus spongiosum	Vestibular bulbs
Proximal shaft of penis	Labia minora
Spongy urethra	Vestibule
Bulbo-urethral glands	Greater vestibular glands
Scrotum	Labia majora

DEVELOPMENT OF FEMALE EXTERNAL GENITALIA

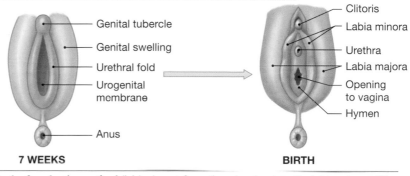

In the female, the urethral folds do not fuse; they develop into the labia minora. The genital swellings will form the labia majora. The genital tubercle develops into the clitoris. The urethra opens to the exterior immediately posterior to the clitoris. The hymen remains as an elaboration of the urogenital membrane.